MONROE COLLEGE LIBRARY

3 7910 01973094 1

WITHDRAWN FROM MONROE COLLEGE LIBRARY

Florence Nightingale and the Nursing Legacy

Second Edition

Building the Foundations of Modern Nursing & Midwifery

By

Monica E. Baly

D0898320

BainBridgeBooks
Philadelphia

RT
81
.G7
B35
1998

Published June 1998 by
BainBridgeBooks
an imprint of
Trans-Atlantic Publications Inc.
Website: www.transatlanticpub.com

ISBN: 1-891696-01-7

Library of Congress Catalog # 98-70738

PRINTED IN THE UNITED STATES OF AMERICA

Second Edition first published in 1997
by Whurr Publishers Ltd
© 1997 By Whurr Publishers
All rights reserved.

No part of this publications may be
reproduced, stored in a retrieval system,
or transmitted in any form or by any
means, electronic, mechanical,
photocopying, recording or otherwise,
without the prior permission of the publisher.

First edition published in 1986 by
Croom Helm Ltd

Contents

To the late Sir Desmond Bonham Carter,
the grandson of Henry Bonham Carter

Preface to the Second Edition

It is ten years since this book was first published and during that time there has been an upsurge of interest in the history of nursing both in Great Britain and abroad. For the past 12 years the History of Nursing Society has been active in the United Kingdom and its journal, an international publication launched in 1995, has provided encouragement and publicity for new research. There has been a burgeoning of interest in Canada[1], Australia[2] and the United States with conferences at national and international level. In Germany and elsewhere in Europe nurses have set an example to us in not suppressing unpalatable facts and realising that it is the truth, not myth, that will make us free.[3] In England the University of Nottingham has organised two successful three-day international conferences on The History of Nursing and Women's History and the Politics of Welfare.[4] In 1989 the International Council of Nurses issued a Mission Statement:

> A study of history and the history of nursing provides an understanding of nursing's past that is critical to assessing present trends and the future of the profession.[5]

In all this debate there has been inevitable discussion and reappraisal of the influence, whether real or imagined, of Florence Nightingale, ranging from those who attribute all the ills nursing has suffered, such as poor pay, harsh discipline and long hours, to her legacy, to those who say that if only she were alive today with her vision, all would be well.

Because more research has been done on nursing and the provision of health care in the nineteenth century we are now better able to see Florence Nightingale in the context of her own time. Studies on nursing care in hospitals before the so-called reforms show that by no means all nurses were drunk and illiterate. Some within the context of their own time were remarkably devoted. Records show that during the cholera epidemic of 1854 the conduct of the nurses was exemplary:

> Sisters showed no concern for themselves, one nurse died having refused
> to report her diarrhoea and go off duty, another developed cholera but
> eventually recovered.

All the nurses and sisters worked without respite, thus earning the unstinted praise of the doctors and governors.[6] A similar story is told in the records at St Bartholomew's in the epidemic of 1847[7] and other hospitals record instances of similar devotion. It must be remembered that as the new regime was forged in the later part of the century many of the old nurses stayed on and gave excellent service. 'The past', as Denis Hay commented, 'is not a Christmas pantomime and seldom, if ever, deals with transformation scenes'.[8]

From about the 1830s it is possible to trace a pattern in the records where the governors were looking for ways to improve their nursing services. First, surgery was getting more ambitious and doctors were looking for more reliable observers; second, the governors with an eye on their subscribers, in what was a fiercely competitive market, were aware that satisfied, grateful patients and success stories brought in the donations. Suggestions for achieving this desired end included appointing a matron with the power 'to keep accounts and to suspend nurses and servants'.[9] There are increasing efforts to bring order into a haphazard system, where although nurses worked inordinate hours, like most workers of the time they came and went much as they pleased, and cooked and ate their meals as best they could. Some hospitals issued rations such as meat, bread, beer or porter, in order to ensure that nurses did not leave the hospital to shop and had less incentive to steal the patients' food. Later many hospitals decided to supply meals ready cooked, and an interesting advisory note to the governors of the Middlesex Hospital adds calculations to show that this would be cheaper for the hospital.[10] Cost analysis is not new.

Keeping the workforce on the premises enabled the authorities to enforce stricter discipline. Reading the registers recording the turnover of nurses one is struck by two factors.

First, there is the high sickness and death rate among nurses.[11] Apart from those who die or who are dismissed as 'not being strong enough for the work' there are those who take fright and leave voluntarily 'for health reasons'. During the first 50 years at the Middlesex Hospital no less than 12 nurses died out of an average complement of eight while at St Bartholomew's in the 1850s–60s 27 nurses died of 'fever'.[11] The cause of death is seldom recorded, but as Florence Nightingale was later to point out, hospitals themselves were a source of infection and did the patient more harm than good.

The second factor is that instant dismissal often seems to be for reasons that today would merely merit a warning. Occasionally a suitable show of repentance brought a reprieve, but dismissal for staying out late, taking a present from a patient or stealing a loaf seems draconian.[12] The reformers made much of the dismissals for 'being found in liquor' in an era when water was contaminated and tea taxed at 100%, and beer and porter were the main drinks available to the poor. Furthermore, in the absence of analgesics – aspirin was not available until 1899 – alcohol and laudanum were the only means of assuaging physical pain or mental distress. Dismissals for insobriety did not cease with the Nightingale reforms nor were they confined to one class of nurses (see Chapter 8).

With a prescience for which credit is seldom given, in the mid-century, governors began to look for the reasons for the high rate of sickness among nurses and came to the conclusion that it was due to long hours and the lack of proper rest periods. This is more than a hundred years before the European Community drafted the Social Chapter and linked overwork with health hazard. Although the hours were reduced, as Helmstadter points out,[13] with the greater control over 'on duty' hours the nurses actually worked harder. The Nightingale nurses worked upwards of a 70-hour week (see p. 204) and although Florence Nightingale tried to insist on nurses having at least eight hours off in 24 and later to be allowed time off for study, she did not seem to think that the hours were excessive.

Contrary to received wisdom nurses were not the lowest paid workers in the nineteenth century. In order to deal with the shortage pay rose steadily even in years of high unemployment. In 1821 a sister at St Bartholomew's earned up to 27 shillings a week and nurses seven shillings.[14] However, as Commissions on Nursing were to find a century or so later, improved pay alone does not bring recruitment; it has to be accompanied by better conditions and status. Being lowly regarded is the greatest disincentive. When nursing became 'fashionable' towards the end of the century it was not because the pay was better or that the conditions were that much improved, but because nursing was seen as being 'respectable'. Nurses were now 'ladies' or, if not, aspired to being thought of as ladies.

The idea that status might be the key to the situation is to be found in mid-century records where doctors and governors suggest that they seek better educated women to supervise the nurses. Inter-hospital conferences are not new. Governors and administrators often consulted one another and the same names appear on different boards. One impetus for this idea was the proliferation of religious communities as a result of the Oxford Movement with its emphasis on the need for the Anglican Church to return to the Catholic tradition and the greater relative importance of good works. This call to women to undertake service by teaching and nursing, especially with the poor, coincided with an imbalance in the ratio of women to men exacerbated by the emigration of many men. Forty-two separate religious communities for women were founded within the Anglican Church between 1845 and 1875.

Florence Nightingale was not the only wealthy, educated woman looking for a purpose in life. Notable among the new nursing orders were the leaders who had provided themselves with some training by visiting hospitals at home and abroad and often by paying for lectures from medical men. The new nursing sisterhoods included St John the Divine, Fitzroy Square, the All Saints Sisters, in Margaret Street, St Margarets, East Grinstead and the Clewer Sisters at Windsor to name but a few around London. Florence Nightingale was wrong when she wrote to Henry Manning, who had just converted to Rome, 'What training is there (in the Church of England) compared with that of a Catholic nun?'.[15] She could have found a vocation within the Church if she had wanted, but her theological speculations at this time show her to be disillusioned with the Church of England.[16]

Apart from Anglican orders there was the growing influence of the Evangelicals with a burgeoning of philanthropic societies of a more Protestant persuasion. Some, like Elizabeth Fry's institute at Bishopsgate and Miss Louise Twining's ladies from St Luke's, Queen's Square, sent suitable acolytes to nearby hospitals to get some nursing experience. There was, therefore, a range of organisations on whom hospitals could call to help improve their nursing service and they consulted with one another as to the best investment. In London, governors made contracts with religious communities for King's College, Charing Cross and University College Hospitals; other hospitals, such as The London, used sisterhoods in times of crisis. The superintendents from such institutions, of all denominations, often had considerable nursing experience and it was in women like Mary Jones and Mother Clare Moore that Florence Nightingale found inspiration when it came to nurse training. As well as staffing some hospitals, trainees from the sisterhoods went to other hospitals, as did Margaret Burt to Guy's, and started a 'reformed' training and organisation.

Contracting nursing out to religious communities undoubtedly improved the standard of nursing, and provided a moral role model and the beginnings of organised training for nurses. However, for hospitals, often on the verge of bankruptcy, there were disadvantages. Because the sisters demanded better conditions and amenities for both patients and staff, the costs rose. When the Westminster Hospital did a cost analysis of the various systems on offer they found that the cheapest way to run a hospital was to keep the work force under the control of the governors and administrators. The bed cost per annum at University College Hospital in the 1880s was £93 9s 5d compared with their own cost of £65 16s 1d. A second disadvantage was that contracting out created an *imperium in imperio*; there were disputes, and the sisters, sometimes backed by the Church militant, were not always tactful (see Chapter 4). When it was suggested to the governors at the Middlesex Hospital that they invite Miss Twining and her ladies to take over the nursing department, they were adamant that nursing must remain under their control. They had probably learnt a lesson from their neighbour in Gower Street. This fear of divided command is probably the reason why it was so difficult to persuade hospitals to accept the Nightingale Fund. Finally, with a spate of defections to Rome, and with one eye on their subscribers, hospitals were fearful that the sisters would proselytise and the governors would be considered 'Romish'. Nevertheless there was a growing body of opinion that the best way to improve the nursing service was to introduce a cadre of better educated women to supervise, and act as mentors to the nurses.

This was not an idea that appealed to Florence Nightingale who was highly critical of her own class, and after the Crimea was even more critical of 'sisterhoods'. She had come to the conclusion that the best nurses:

> Came not from persons of superior manners and education. Ladies in fact are not as a rule required, but rather women of somewhat more ordinary intelligence belonging to women who are habitually employed earning their own living.[17]

In 1860 she gave her considered opinion to Mr Rathbone who was planning a regime for nurses:

> Her [the nurse's] time ought to be fully occupied by her ward work, her necessary sleep and exercise and what making and mending she has to do for herself.[18]

At this stage there is no suggestion that the nurse should have leisure for other pursuits or time for study.

However, after about eight years when it was revealed to her that 'The chief trainer at St Thomas's was a drinking woman' and that, with the exception of Agnes Jones, the Fund had not produced a single woman fit to be a trainer, she reluctantly changed her mind and allowed the recruitment of 'Special Probationers' (usually paying). By this time a number of other teaching hospitals were doing the same.

It is against this background that we must look at the negotiations of St Thomas's with the Nightingale Fund Council in 1860 (see

Chapter 2). St Thomas's had no doubt read the articles in *The Lancet* and had consulted other hospitals and they were determined to avoid a cuckoo in *their* nest. They insisted that the School must be under the control of their matron and the present sisters. It was not what Florence Nightingale herself had envisaged, but she gave in and this accounts for her comment:

> It will be a beginning in a humble way... at least it will not be a beginning with failure, i.e. the possibility of upsetting a large hospital.

St Thomas's had no intention of being upset. Second, there was no danger that the School would put up the costs, the 'wily fox' of a treasurer saw to that. A cursory study of the figures on pp. 39–40 and the timetable for the probationers (see p. 48) will show that the Fund was subsidising the hospital. St Thomas's had a bargain. Finally there was the advantage that the School was secular: there was no fear of subscribers being put off by stories of 'Romish plots'. This was a factor not lost on Miss Nightingale.

What was to become known as the 'Nightingale system' soon became acceptable to other hospitals, even without a subsidy from the Fund. Probationers were cheap, and Lady Probationers even cheaper. The hospital kept control of the work force and could impose a strict contract on the nurses while, at the same time, gaining prestige by virtue of its improved nursing service, now necessary to meet the demands of medicine and the expectations of the middle classes who were starting to use the voluntary hospitals. The 'system' was not of Miss Nightingale's devising; it was forced on her.

No new profession was forged but rather the old one was hastened along the old grooves. Fundamental questions not asked (although Florence Nightingale herself knew these better than most people) included:

- what were the main health needs of the population?
- how could the nurse be trained to meet those needs?
- who should train and educate her?
- how should she be tested and examined?

In spite of this failure there were undoubted improvements in nursing by the end of the century but they must be seen in a constellation of other factors, such as advances in medicine, the better education of women, the lack of opportunity for women elsewhere and the women's movement itself, changed attitude of the public to doctors and hospitals and, above all, what we would now call 'media coverage' which depicted the nurse as a 'ministering angel'.

Before we are critical of the Nightingale legacy it is worth asking this question: Given the economic plight of hospitals, the position of women, and the social conditions of the period, how else, or where else, could nurses have been trained in 1860?

No one knew better than Florence Nightingale that the health needs of the population were *outside* the hospital, but it would take nearly another hundred years before training and education could be planned for nurses to meet the total needs of the population.

In history what happened is often the only thing that could have happened, given the circumstances of the time.

Notes

1. Baly, M.E., The Canadian first National Conference. *History of Nursing Journal,* vol. 2, no. 6, p. 47, 1988.
2. Blewitt, N., Opening address, History of Nursing Conference, Australia 1993. Ibid., vol. 4, no. 6, p. 259.
3. Steppe, H., Nursing in the Third Reich. Ibid. vol. 3, no. 4, p. 21. See also *International History of Nursing Journal,* vol. 1, no. 4, 1996.
4. McGann, S. and Nuttall, P., Nottingham Women's History and the Politics of Welfare. Ibid. vol. 4, no. 6, p. 330.
5. International Council of Nurses Congress Report 1989, reported in *History of Nursing Journal,* vol. 3, no. 1, editorial.
6. Board of Governors' Minutes, Middlesex Hospital, September 1854.
7. Yeo, G., *Nursing at Barts* (Alan Sutton Publishing, 1995).
8. Hay, D., *Italian Renaissance* (Cambridge University Press, Cambridge, 1970), p. 2.
9. Collins, S., Victorian matrons at the London. *History of Nursing Journal,* vol. 15, no. 2, p. 57.
   Helmstadter, C., Nurse recruitment and retention in C19th London teaching hospitals. *History of Nursing Journal,* vol. 2, no. 1, 1996.
10. BL, Add Mss 45752, f. 126f.
11. Yeo, G., ibid., p. 25.
12. Board of Governors' Minutes, Middlesex Hospital, 1750–1800, ibid., April 1850.
13. Helmstadter, C., *History of Nursing Journal,* vol. 2, no. 1, 1996.
14. Yeo, G., ibid., p. 22.
15. Nightingale, F. and Manning, H., July 1852, St Mary of the Angels, Wellcome Institute photocopy.
16. Baly, M.E., *'As Miss Nightingale Said... '* 2nd edn (Baillière Tindall, London, 1997), Chapter 3.
17. Mayhew, P., *All Saints: The Birth and Growth of a Community* (Parchment, Oxford, 1989).
18. Nightingale, F./Rathbone W., BL, Add Mss 47753, June 1860, ff. 1–4.

Acknowledgements

The first edition of this book arose out of the research undertaken on behalf of the Nightingale Fund Council and I acknowledge the help given by Lady Bonham Carter, at that time secretary to the Fund Council, and by the late Sir Desmond Bonham Carter and especially for Sir Desmond's recollections of his great-grandfather, Henry Bonham Carter, without whose hoarding of Florence Nightingale's vast epistolary output on nursing much of the material on which this book was based would have been lost. My thanks are also due to Professor W. F. Bynum of the Wellcome Institute for the History of Medicine who supervised my research and encouraged me when the sheer quantity of material seemed overwhelming, and to the late, and sadly missed, Professor Brian Abel-Smith who read the script and sent the quintessential Abel-Smith comment, 'Thank God the telephone had not been invented then.'

During my research I had help from a number of librarians, particularly Mrs Howlett at the Greater London Record Office, the staff at the British Library, the librarians at St Thomas's Hospital and the Earl of Pembroke who allowed me to read the relevant Herbert papers at Wilton House. I would also like to record my thanks to the Canadian Nurses Association for their valuable help with Chapter 8 and to Dr Anne Summers for reading and advising on the chapter on military nursing. During my attempts to make some comparison between early training schools in the nineteenth century and to trace the Nightingale nurses who went to the Middlesex Hospital, I was helped by the late Dr Ralph Winterton, the archivist there at that time, whose notes on nursing in the nineteenth century at the hospital were invaluable.

Since 1986 I have come to realise that we cannot understand Florence Nightingale's attitude to health unless we understand her personal and idiosyncratic religion. First, I had to understand the central message in those three volumes known, as *Suggestions for Thought* that Strachey called her 'metaphysical disquisitions' with their convoluted prose and subjunctive clauses. In comprehending them I am grateful to prebendary Richard Askew, the rector of Bath Abbey, for his interest and advice on my attempts to summarise the endless Victorian theological debates.

I also owe a debt to Susan McGann, the archivist for the Royal College of Nursing, who directed me to that delightful sketch opposite of Florence Nightingale done by Lord Cadogan in 1856 in the Crimea and, of course, to his great-grandson, Mr J.S. Brichiere-Colombi, who gave us permission to use it.

Monica E. Baly
Bath 1997

The portrait of Florence Nightingale, which is signed by her, was painted on 14 May 1856 by Colonel (Later General) Sir George Cadogan of the Grenadier Guards who was the Queen's Commissioner to the Sardinian Army in the Crimea. After the Crimean War he was the Military Attaché to the British Embassy in Florence where his daughter, Lady Sophia Cadogan, married the Marchese Augusto Brichieri-Colombi. The portrait is from George Cadogan's Crimea Sketchbook *which includes many battles and scenes of military life in the Crimea. It is now on loan to the National Army Museum and the portrait is reproduced with kind permission of Mr J.S. Brichieri-Colombi.*

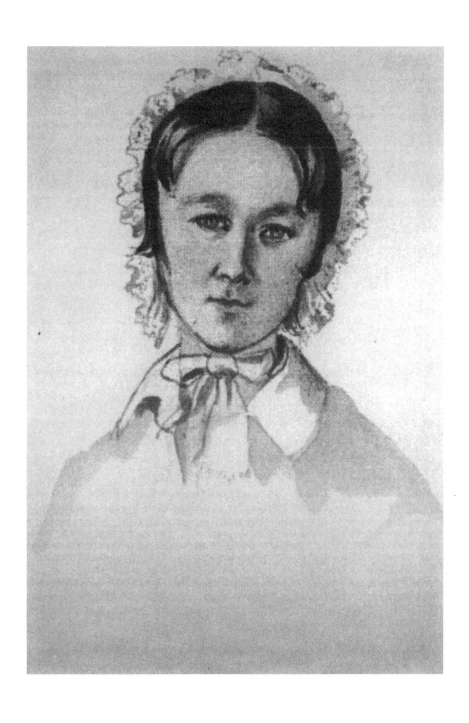

Introduction

This book is based on the archive material belonging to the Nightingale Fund Council and other records associated with the work of the Fund between 1855 and 1914. Although the work of the Fund Council continues to this day, after the death of Miss Nightingale in 1910 and the introduction of a three-year training at St Thomas's, it ceased to play a decisive role. The pioneering days were over.

This material sheds a new light on the early Nightingale schools and their influence which, for a variety of reasons, has been overlooked by general historians and unexplored, or ignored, by nurse historians. Because Miss Nightingale's life was so long, her work so varied and her character a source of perennial fascination, general historians have given little attention to the nursing achievement. Sir Edward Cook's seminal study was concerned with the life of Miss Nightingale as a whole[1] and nursing finds a comparatively small place in his two volumes. In preparing his work Sir Edward consulted Henry Bonham Carter who was not only Miss Nightingale's cousin and her executor but also still the secretary of the Nightingale Fund. Henry was a lawyer and in 1909 some of the characters from the earlier nursing scene were still alive, or only recently dead, and with interested relatives watching their reputations. Besides such legal and personal considerations there was the delicate question of the current relationship of St Thomas's hospital and the Nightingale Fund with the hospital authorities still driving a hard bargain. Moreover, although nurse training was now generally accepted it was still necessary to hammer home the message, and Henry Bonham Carter had a vested interest in a success story. In Cook's 'Life' the rough places were made smooth and no turbulence ruffles the waters.

Because Cook's work is so monumental most other studies since have been a recension of it. Mrs Woodham-Smith uses some new material[2] but as far as nursing is concerned she relies heavily on Cook, and the fact that she later contemplated writing another book on

1

nursing indicates that she was aware of this lack. However, when asked by the Fund Council to research the papers and produce a history of the Fund she declined. In turn many other historians have relied on Woodham-Smith – or Cook via Woodham-Smith – and even those like Professor Barry Smith who have sought to break the hagiographical approach have fallen into the trap of quoting from Cook as far as nursing is concerned.[3]

Two examples illustrate the danger of this approach. Cook, no doubt prompted by Henry Bonham Carter, whose remembrance of things past may have been patchy, gives two reasons for the choice of St Thomas's: that it was rich, large and well managed – which in 1859 it was not – and that the matron was 'a woman after Miss Nightingale's own heart – strong, devoted to her work, devoid of all self-seeking, full of decision and administrative ability'.[4] In order to support this Cook quotes from the obituary article on Mrs Wardroper that Miss Nightingale wrote in her best panegyric style some 32 years later which includes the much-quoted phrase 'she never went a-pleasuring, seldom into society'.[5] However, during the intervening years there are dozens of letters which show that far from finding Mrs Wardroper 'full of decision and administrative ability' Miss Nightingale and Henry Bonham Carter spent long hours striving to save Mrs Wardroper from herself, complaining that she 'acted like an insane king by divine right' and, more and more, seeking to take the training school out of her hands. But every subsequent biographer, including Barry Smith, has implied that Mrs Wardroper was the moving force and 'she educated her [Miss Nightingale] in nursing matters'.[6] Almost all biographers, without exception, quote from the obituary notice as if it represented Miss Nightingale's opinion in 1860. Historians would do well too to remember Dr Johnson's dictum that 'in lapidary inscriptions a man is not on oath'.

The second and almost universally quoted myth is that the new St Thomas's at Lambeth was Miss Nightingale's choice and in the battle over the new site she got her way. Fifty years later Henry Bonham Carter probably did not wish to disclose that Miss Nightingale had been worsted, nor did he wish to recall that she had referred to this imposing edifice on the banks of the Thames as being 'on the worst site in London'. This is important because Miss Nightingale used St Thomas's for her School because she thought it would be moved to the suburbs, and when her advice was ignored one of the main reasons for her choice had gone, which coloured her relationship with St Thomas's and its officers in the 1870s. History has proved Miss Nightingale right. For the next 60 years or more report after report complained that there were too many hospitals in London.

Had Miss Nightingale's advice been taken and the map in *Notes on Hospitals*[7] heeded much of the present trauma following the Tomlinson report would have been avoided.[8]

One of the most popular legends is that the Nightingale School was immediately successful and that thanks to a rigorous training, lectures, supervision and constant assessment the probationers were models of decorum, most becoming superintendents and missionaries for the School. To quote Mrs Woodham-Smith 'Neat, lady-like, vestal, above suspicion she [the probationer] must be the incarnate denial that the hospital nurse need be drunken, ignorant and promiscuous.'[9]

Here Mrs Woodham-Smith is following Cook and subsequent biographers. All refer to the monthly reports, the diary keeping and the instruction received from the sisters, but they do not mention that Miss Nightingale soon found the monthly report meaningless and that few probationers kept diaries, those who did showing that they received little instruction. No one refers to the high wastage rate, the ill health and the dismissals for misconduct – including dismissals for insobriety. The beloved anecdotes of probationers trekking to visit Miss Nightingale refer to the mid-1870s or later, and not to the early years.

Perhaps one of the most misleading myths is that the Nightingale School was unique because it was 'independent'. Lucy Seymer writes: 'the distinctive advance made by the Nightingale School was due to its independence. From the first its liberal endowment has allowed it to hold fast to its educational ideals.'[10] It is true that the Fund's school was more independent in the secular field than anything that had gone before inasmuch as the Fund paid for the maintenance of 15 probationers and money towards the salary of the matron and the Resident Medical Officer to give instruction. But the Fund Council could not check the ability to teach nor could it ensure that instruction was given. The probationers were assistant nurses and used by the hospital as staff and Miss Nightingale was soon to bewail that they were merely 'doing the hospital's work'. Try as they might the Council never succeeded in persuading the hospital authorities to give regular and reasonable time off for lectures or special instruction for those destined to be superintendents.

As the nature of the hospital changed authorities were not slow to see the value of disciplined, biddable probationers used as assistant nurses and, as more nurses were needed, so matrons were pressed to take on more probationers, more than Miss Nightingale thought there was scope for training. At St Thomas's this meant that the Fund contributed an increasingly small proportion to the cost and the School grew progressively less 'independent'.

In spite of the increase in the number of probationers by the end of the nineteenth century the number of trained nurses was comparatively small compared with the need. Professor Abel-Smith points out: 'it is unlikely that there were more than 10,000 nurses whose training would have satisfied Miss Nightingale. The number who were ladies and trained was probably less than 5,000.'[11] Therefore, after 40 years, far from 'the hospital world being revolutionised by educated refined women' as Lavinia Dock claimed,[12] they represented a comparatively small proportion of nurses. Indeed by the end of the century many trained nurses quickly left hospital for the freer world of private nursing. Nevertheless 'ladies and trained' represented the leadership and it was the leadership that produced authors of textbooks and histories of nursing. Anxious to portray nursing as a homogeneous, educated profession, to be publicised as such, they tended to exaggerate the revolution, overstating what they called the Sairy Gamp era and ignoring the progress made by nursing institutions in the middle of the nineteenth century. The early histories like to portray the Nightingale reforms as a dramatic break with the past. But there was no sudden beam from Miss Nightingale's lamp; reform came slowly and painfully and what became known as the Nightingale system was not an ideal scheme of Miss Nightingale's devising but pragmatic experiment and the result of enforced compromise. The compromise between the hospital authorities who wanted to use probationers as pairs of hands, the doctors who wished to keep nurses accountable to them, and the Council who wished to instigate a system of planned training with nurses accountable to trained nurses gave the twentieth century its nursing legacy.

Notes

1. Cook, Sir E., *The Life of Florence Nightingale*, 2 vols (Macmillan, London, 1913).
2. Woodham-Smith, C., *Florence Nightingale* (Constable, London, 1950).
3. Smith, F.B., *Florence Nightingale – Reputation and Power* (Croom Helm, London & Canberra, 1982).
4. Cook, *The Life of Florence Nightingale*, vol. 1, p. 458.
5. *British Medical Journal*, 31 December 1892.
6. Smith, *Florence Nightingale*, p. 348.
7. Nightingale, F., *Notes on Hospitals* 3rd edn. (Longmans Green & Co, London, 1863) (for a reproduction of the map see Baly, M., *As Miss Nightingale Said...* Scutari, London, 1991, p. 52–53)

8. Department of Health and Education (1992) *Report of the Inquiry into London's Health Services Medical Education and Research* (Tomlinson Report) (HMSO, London).

9. Woodham-Smith, *Florence Nightingale,* p. 348.

10. Seymer, L.R., *A General History of Nursing* (Faber and Faber, London, 1960), p. 96.

11. Abel-Smith, B., *A History of the Nursing Profession* (Heinemann, London, 1960), p. 57.

12. Dock, L., and Stewart, I.S., *A Short History of Nursing,* 4th edn (Putman's Sons, London & New York, 1920), p. 126.

1. The Nightingale Fund

It now becomes the duty of the public to show her that her services have been and are duly appreciated in this country... and how that honour, which is her due, can be paid to her in the manner most grateful and most agreeable to her...

HRH the Duke of Cambridge, 29 November 1855

In October 1854 William Howard Russell, the war correspondent to *The Times* in the Crimea, sent back his famous vitriolic despatches to England in which he complained of the incompetence and muddle in the prosecution of the war and in particular the lack of hospital provision with dressers and nurses. Why have we no Sisters of Charity?, asked *The Times*.[1]

Much of the public indignation that followed fell on the head of Sidney Herbert who was Minister at War and responsible for its financial administration, and who was suspected of dragging his feet because his mother was a Russian.[2] On 15 October Sidney Herbert wrote to Miss Nightingale, whom he knew well, and who was nursing in Harley Street at the Institution for the Care of Sick Gentlewomen, and asked her to take a party of nurses at the government's expense to Scutari.[3] Miss Nightingale agreed and hastily assembled a party of 38 nurses consisting of 14 professional nurses and 24 others, including five Bermondsey nuns and 14 from Anglican orders.

The expedition reached Scutari on 5 November and climbed the slopes to the Turkish barracks to the gateway over which Miss Nightingale said should have been written Dante's words: 'All hope abandon, ye who enter here.' The barracks, which were serving as a base hospital, were filthy, dilapidated and had no sanitation. To make matters worse the party was received with sullen opposition and the doctors refused the help offered by the nurses. Miss Nightingale was patient and used the enforced waiting period to spend some of the money raised by private subscription, of which she had charge, to buy much needed supplies and press various people into service.[4] Then on 9 November with the battle of Balaclava the situation changed and the sick and wounded began to pour across the Bosphorus; as the hospital filled, so the doctors turned to Miss Nightingale for help.

For the next six months Miss Nightingale and her party battled against overwhelming odds, not only nursing four miles of patients, but reorganising the cooking arrangements, purveying much of the hospital, organising repairs and arranging for the welfare of the wounded. There was still some hostility to the experiment and the situation was fraught with internal antagonisms, but Miss Nightingale's letters home and despatches to Sidney Herbert, if somewhat exaggerated,[5] were read with interest as were the glowing accounts from wounded soldiers. Queen Victoria took an interest in the work of Miss Nightingale and her nurses, and sent despatches to the wounded soldiers and personal messages to Miss Nightingale herself.[6] By the spring the Nightingale nurses had become a legend and Miss Nightingale a popular heroine.

In May of 1855 the conditions in the barracks hospital had so improved that Miss Nightingale was able to cross to the Crimea and inspect the hospitals there. Within a week or so of her arrival she was struck down by Crimean fever and was seriously ill. Attended by Mr Bracebridge, an old friend who had accompanied her to Scutari, Mrs Roberts, one of her nurses, and Private Robinson and Private Thomas, she eventually recovered; the crisis passed and the news, telegraphed to England by Lord Raglan, was the subject of general thanksgiving. Queen Victoria wrote to Lord Panmure, now Secretary for War, that she was 'truly thankful to learn that that excellent and valuable person Miss Nightingale is safe'.[7]

The unique characteristic of the Crimean war was not that its cause carried little conviction, that its administration was inefficient or that its army was ill equipped; thanks to the telegraph the story could be sent day by day to appear at British breakfast tables within a day or two. The public took the good news with the bad. The news of Miss Nightingale's recovery was good. After the terrible losses of the battle of Balaclava, the disastrous winter followed by an outcry in the press, the Aberdeen administration had fallen, and Palmerston had become Prime Minister, but as yet the management of the war gave no cause for rejoicing. Of the 97,800 men who took the field 2,700 had been killed, 1,800 had died of wounds while a staggering 17,600 had died of disease.[8] Bad though these figures were, letters and accounts from soldiers suggested they would have been worse but for the ministration of Miss Nightingale and her nurses. Their assumption was probably right because our French allies lost 24 per cent of their army from disease, and the Russian army was almost halved from this cause.[9]

Miss Nightingale had become a national heroine and the Nightingale family were inundated with gifts – suitable and unsuitable – to be sent to her for the comfort of the wounded. There was also a suggestion that there should be some kind of public testimonial which her sister, Parthe, described as the 'bracelet and tea pot kind'. Referring to this wave of emotion later Sidney Herbert said:

> There broke out in different parts of the country a feeling of immediate and spontaneous expression of public gratitude to her and isolated portions of the community were organising committees and preparing to make gifts to her – we felt it was right to give appropriate direction to this generous feeling.[10]

Mrs Carter Hall, whose husband was well known in hospital circles, had the idea of collecting from the women of England, but on discussing the matter with Mrs Sidney Herbert, who was a close friend of Miss Nightingale, it was decided to enlarge the scheme to a national appeal. Mrs Herbert and the Nightingale family were sure that Miss Nightingale would refuse any personal tribute and the only object for which an appeal would be acceptable would be one that would enable her to carry out some public service near to her heart. Perhaps, it was suggested, she might like to form an English Kaiserwerth, and the matter was eventually put to Miss Nightingale herself now back in Scutari.

Before she went to the Crimea Miss Nightingale had considered the possibility of taking an appointment as superintendent of the rebuilt King's College Hospital. Medical men had been impressed with her organising ability at Harley Street and Mr William Bowman, a surgeon at King's College, pressed her strongly.[11] While she was still at Harley Street Miss Nightingale also became friendly with Dr Bence Jones of St George's who had ideas about introducing a training school for nurses at that hospital and she was interested. But in 1854 Miss Nightingale went to Scutari. In August 1855 Dr Bence Jones wrote to Miss Nightingale in the Crimea to express his joy at her recovery and he went on to solicit her help with his plans for a training school for nurses. The main point of his plan was that the governors should make nurse training one of their objectives and they should appoint a super-intendent

> with no ward to take care of but who shall specially direct and instruct persons being trained... and that persons admitted for training should be lodged within the hospital and obey certain rules... the object being scarcely inferior to the education of a medical man.[12]

Dr Bence Jones clearly had in mind that eventually all teaching hospitals should start training schools and employ separately recruited tutors. Unfortunately Miss Nightingale's reply is not available, but it accounts for a statement in her reply to Sidney Herbert on 29 September 1855 when he wrote and asked her to provide a plan for the use of the Nightingale Fund: 'Dr Bence Jones has written to me for a plan for St George's. People seem to think that I have nothing to do but to sit here and make plans.'[13] In other words everyone was asking her about plans for the future but with the fighting still going on she had something else to think about. However, although she was not enthusiastic about a Fund, she was interested enough, and astute enough, to add a caveat that she must be allowed full control of the money. In Scutari Miss Nightingale had learned the hard way the fate of those who handle funds where the control is ambiguous.

Notwithstanding this cool reply, a provisional committee was set up with Sidney Herbert and Samuel Carter Hall as joint secretaries, Sidney Herbert having left the War Office in January. Even before Miss Nightingale replied it looks as if there were plans afoot for a national appeal as early as August because there is a letter from Sidney Herbert to Carter Hall asking that 'a Fund circular be prepared to be sent to 300 banking houses'.[14]

In November 1855 the provisional committee, which consisted of 70 distinguished persons including Lord Panmure, the Speaker of the House and the Lord Chief Justice, took the lease of the first-floor chambers in 5 Parliament Street for a year.[15] On 8 November, with Sidney Herbert in the chair, a meeting of the committee was called to agree certain resolutions to be presented to a national meeting at which it was intended to launch the national appeal. These resolutions were important because they are the basis on which the money was given and on which the subsequent Deeds of Trust were drawn up. They were:

1. The noble exertions of Miss Nightingale in the hospitals of the East demand the grateful recognition of the British people.
2. That while it is known that Miss Nightingale would decline any such recognition merely personal to herself it is understood that she will accept it in a form that may enable her, on her return to England, to establish a permanent institution for the training, sustenance and protection of nurses and to arrange for their proper instruction and employment in metropolitan hospitals [metropolitan was deleted at a subsequent meeting].
3. That to accomplish this object on a scale worthy of the nation and honourable to Miss Nightingale herself, a public subscription be opened to which all classes be invited to contribute and application

be made for the 'red' of the clergy, the mayors of corporate towns and other available sources of assistance.

4. That the sums thus collected be applied to these objects according to the discretion of Miss Nightingale and under regulations formed by herself, the subscribers having entire confidence in her tried energy and judgement.[16]

The following week the Committee added to Resolution 4:

... and in the meantime Trustees shall be considered protectors of the Fund.

The Committee then set in motion the calling of a public meeting at Willis's Rooms in King's Street off St James's Square for Thursday, 29 November, and an invitation to the Duke of Cambridge, the Commander-in-Chief of the army, to take the chair. The Duke, an admirer of Miss Nightingale, accepted and the meeting was planned to have 100 persons on the platform and to issue a further 1,250 tickets. In the event the room proved too small and it was suffocating; nevertheless it was described by *The Times* as 'Brilliant, enthusiastic and harmonious'. The composite resolution was moved by the Duke of Argyll and seconded by the Hon. and Reverend Sydney Godolphin Osborne, a volunteer chaplain who had assisted Miss Nightingale in Scutari. A second resolution was put forward by Lord Goderich – Prime Minister briefly in 1827 – seconded by the Reverend Dr Cumming, and moved that Miss Nightingale be asked to name a Council and that the Rt Hon. Sidney Herbert and Samuel Carter Hall, Esq. continue as secretaries to the Fund. Lord Stanley, the Duke of Argyll, and Sidney Herbert – all of whom had been associated with the prosecution of the war – made speeches. However, it was probably Richard Monckton Milnes who captured the imagination of the audience by comparing (with poetic licence excusing geographical inaccuracy) the glittering scene in St James's with

the scene which met the gaze of that noble woman who was now devoting herself to the service of her suffering fellow creatures on the black shores of Crim Tartary overlooking the waters of the inhospitable sea.[17]

A copy of the proceedings of the meeting was sent to Miss Nightingale and in the meantime the Earl of Ellesmere, the Rt Hon. Sidney Herbert, the Rt Hon. Stuart Wortley, Sir William Heathcote, Richard Monckton Milnes, Charles H. Mills and Charles H. Bracebridge were appointed as Trustees of the Fund. One of the first tasks of the Trustees was to send a deputation to wait on the Lord

Mayor at the Mansion House. The result of this deputation was the setting up of the Auxiliary Committee for the City with the Lord Mayor as treasurer and a meeting of the leading merchants and bankers of the City was called for 19 December. The Committee was to give the Trustees some problems and subsequent events showed that it was neither the source of help nor the cornucopia of wealth that had been hoped.

By Christmas 1855 20,000 circulars had been despatched,[18] mostly to mayors and the beneficed clergy but also including some 5,000 to minor dissenting bodies and 3,000 to Roman Catholics. From this circulation the Fund received, or was promised, £7,000. A Finance Committee was then formed with Lord Monteagle, who had known Miss Nightingale since childhood, as chairman; the other members were John Thornton, Robert Biddulph, of the firm of Cocks and Biddulph, and Edward Marjoribanks, of Coutts, another old friend of Miss Nightingale who she said had taught her all she knew about accounts.

In January 1856 Sidney Herbert received Miss Nightingale's official reply. It was gracious but not enthusiastic, and taken in conjunction with her private comments it is clear that Miss Nightingale did not see the Fund as an unmixed blessing:

Dear Mr Herbert,

In answer to your letter proposing the undertaking of a Training School for Nurses I will beg to say that it is impossible for me to express what I have felt in regard to the sympathy and confidence shown to me by the originators and supporters of the scheme. Exposed as I am to misinterpreted and misunderstood in a field of action in which the work is new and complicated, distant from many who sit judgement upon it, it is indeed an abiding support to have such sympathy and such appreciation brought home to me in the midst of labour and difficulties all but overpowering. I must add however that while the pressure of work is such that I would never desert for any other, so long as I see room to believe that what I do here is unfinished, I am very doubtful if they continue it will leave me life and health for the work I am asked to undertake. May I then beg you to express to the Committee that I accept their proposal provided I may do so on the understanding of this great uncertainty and whether it will ever be possible for me to carry it out. In such uncertainty I feel it irrelevant to appoint a Council to represent me, and I would far rather leave such funds as may be collected in the hands of yourself and Mr Bracebridge relieving you however of some responsibility in the case of my death by naming the following to decide on the mode of employing the money in conjunction with yourselves – which money as far as I am concerned I should then wish to be left free to be employed on any benevolent object approved by you.

Lord Ellesmere   The Dean of Hereford
Col. Jebb   Sir J. McNeill
Sir James Clark   Dr Bence Jones
Mr Wm. Bowman

With regard to the General Committee I thank my friends for making additions to it which I might suggest but I am perfectly satisfied with it as is stands.

Believe me to be,
yours very truly
Florence Nightingale[19]

It will be noted that out of a Council of nine, four were eminent doctors. For one whose aim was to wrest power from doctors in nursing matters, and who wrote to Sidney Herbert 'as for doctors military and civil there must be something in the smell of medicine which includes administrative incapacity',[20] the proportion seems rather high.

None of the Council knew what Miss Nightingale meant by nurse training, and indeed at this stage her own ideas were by no means clear. She had looked at nurse training all over Europe and at the schemes that were springing up in England under the aegis of religious movements; she discussed endlessly the merits and demerits of each system, but to her they were all flawed. Apart from the sectarian antagonisms surrounding religious orders their training was unscientific and, in Miss Nightingale's eyes an even greater sin, it was usually unhygienic. With good reason she was disenchanted with 'lady nurses' who would not have the stamina for 'such laborious work'. What Miss Nightingale wanted was a system that would synthesise the best of the moral purpose of the religious orders but would be non-sectarian, the educational background of the upper middle classes and the hardihood of working-class women. She knew this synthesis would be hard to achieve and would only come with years of trial and error.[21]

The way she was thinking at this time is reflected in a letter sent to Mrs Bracebridge at the same time as her official reply to Sidney Herbert. Mrs Bracebridge had obviously asked her about her plans for the Fund. 'I have no plan', she writes and goes on to say:

There is no certainty of failure more complete than the idea of beginning anything of the nature proposed with a great demonstration... if I had a plan it would simply be to take the poorest and least organised hospital in London and, putting myself there, see what I could do – not touching the Fund for years till experience had shown how the Fund might best be available. This is not to detract from the value of the Fund to the work. It will be invaluable as the occasion arises.[22]

Apart from the pressure of work in the Crimea Miss Nightingale had other reservations about tying herself to being the superintendent of some institution when she returned home. She had, through her unique position and her own acute intelligence, gained a great deal of knowledge about the workings, and failings, of the Army Medical Service such as the regimental system and the methods of purveying which she determined to put right. There is probably a grain of truth in Professor Smith's assertion that 'having tasted power she was determined to use it'.[23] Given to dramatic but telling statements she said, 'I stand at the altar of murdered men' and the task of ensuring that never again did the British army suffer a 73 per cent mortality in six months was to be her priority.

During the eight months between the meeting in Willis's Rooms and Miss Nightingale's return to England in July 1856, the Nightingale Fund had a large and distinguished Committee, a Council appointed by Miss Nightingale herself (see letter above), Trustees in whose names the money was invested and various sub-committees to deal with different aspects of fund raising. By June 1856 the Fund stood at £32,000 but this had been achieved by dint of much hard work and anxiety on the part of the Committee as the letters which passed almost daily between the two secretaries testify. The Fund was not taken up quite as 'heartily' as has been suggested.[24]

The short notice at which meetings were arranged and the alacrity with which circulars were printed, collected and sent out seem incredible even in the age of information technology. Public meetings were put on in Leeds, Manchester, Glasgow, Oxford, Bath, Brighton and many other places. Getting the right man for the right place was always a problem. In January 1856 Sidney Herbert was writing to Carter Hall: '... have we a Committee man who could go to Oxford or Leeds? Monckton Milnes would be good on resolutions but what about Gladstone?'[25] There were plenty of suggestions about places that should be canvassed and who should be approached. Many of Sidney Herbert's replies have been preserved from which it can be deduced that he was inundated with advice and that he must surely have needed that angelic temperament that Miss Nightingale was later to ascribe to him.

Much thought was given to getting publicity. W.H. Smith placed 1,000 leaflets containing the objectives of the Fund at the railway stations with which he was connected. *The Times*, whose editor, John Delane, was a friend of the Nightingale family, carried a number of articles, full reports of meetings and the subscription lists. Articles written by Sidney Herbert himself, or with a poetic dash by Monckton Milnes appeared in the various weekly journals. In March Jenny Lind

(Madam Goldschmidt) gave a concert in the Exeter Hall which was a brilliant occasion giving the Fund not only £1,872 5s 0d but also some useful publicity.[26]

No time was wasted: the Committee met weekly in their rooms in Parliament Street, letters were sent out on Christmas Eve and meetings held on 27 December; Sidney Herbert wrote from Reading station, on the way to a Fund meeting, 'I avail myself of a delay between trains here to send you the note Lord Monteagle required in order for Coutts to finalise exchequer bills.'[27] But the organisational worries of the Committee were as nothing compared with the religious and sectarian bickerings with which they were beset. Almost as soon as the Fund was launched trouble began, Sidney Herbert writing, 'There has been a silly attack on Miss Nightingale in the press, but no one who knows Miss Nightingale can entertain suspicions of her on religious grounds.'[28] In January 1856 he wrote:

> I will now want a public meeting to get rid of all the idle and foolish objections that are started against the scheme. The article in the *Herald* is written in ignorance of our plan since what it recommends us to do, and blames me for not doing, is the one thing we are doing... Other members of the Committee would do better than I. I am supposed to have High Church leanings and a Low Church certificate would not be much value. Perhaps Monckton Milnes or Sydney Osborne would be best...[29]

As soon as he had Miss Nightingale's reply Sidney Herbert got a favourable article in *The Times* disclaiming that the Fund was linked with any religious group, but in spite of this he complains that the meeting at Manchester was troubled by religious bigotry and that some were under the impression that Miss Nightingale 'was almost an R.C.'. On another occasion, when the Bishop of Oxford asked for a meeting to be postponed, Sidney Herbert wrote that it was too late and he was writing to the Bishop of Lincoln or Ripon: 'It is important to have a Bishop to counteract the charge of Socinianism that has been levelled at Miss Nightingale and the charge of Romanism by Dr Cummings, the Presbyterian.'[30]

The fervour with which the religious question was pursued runs through the letters and indicates that most people expected nursing reform to come through some quasi-religious order, perhaps on the lines of the order under Miss Sellon and the Bishop of Exeter at Devonport. As many of the nursing sisterhoods were linked with the Anglican Church and the Oxford Movement, the Nonconformists had the most to fear, and this is why Manchester and the City of London were particularly difficult. To a country divided over the disestablishment of the Church, its reform and the preachings of the Oxford Movement as opposed to Methodism it is small wonder that supporters of different religious sects wanted to be sure that their money was not going to a rival concern. The heavy emphasis that the Fund Council put on its non-sectarian aims accounts for the insistence that the nursing school must be based on a secular authority, even though members like Sidney Herbert and William Bowman might personally have wished for a link with the sisters of St John.[31]

Besides the religious questions there were political crosscurrents. Of the politicians who helped with the Fund and donated generously it is noticeable that there was a higher ratio among those who had criticised the conduct of the war. On the other hand the sharpest comment came from the radicals, who tended to be Nonconformists and suspicious of the way the Fund might be used. Again, although Sidney Herbert was popular, he had been a staunch Peelite and was therefore suspect in the eyes of some landowners because of his support for free trade. It is clear that there was a political background because there are letters from supporters or collectors saying they are 'the wrong political colour' for their area.[32]

One persistent problem that beset the Council when appealing for money was that they could give no clear indication as to how the money would be applied. Miss Nightingale had persistently written that she had no plans for the Fund and, with some justification, had said in a covering letter:

> It would have been reasonable to have asked for a prospectus of my plans if I had originally *asked* for the money, which of course I did not. But to furnish a cut and dried prospectus of my plans, situated as I am here when I cannot look forward to a month, much less a year is what I would not if I could, and could not if I would.[33]

This is a typically logical, if acerbic, Nightingale comment which, although printed in *The Times,* did not help the Council.

Two of the main sources of subscription were the armed services and the Church. The first Sunday in May was declared Thanksgiving Day, and many a clergyman adapted his sermon accordingly. The Vicar of Ballygawley in Ireland wrote: 'I explained to my people the work of Miss Nightingale and what I send you is exclusively the offering of the poor; I have no rich man in my parish.'[34]

The story from many parishes is the same. A parish in Cornwall collected 3s 6d 'and would do more if they could see the need'. That they did not see the need was hardly surprising; few parishioners would have seen a hospital and most were brought up in the tradition that families were responsible for their own sick. The story from the parishes in the north is a sad comment on the precarious state of employment in 1856.

The Fund was notified to the army in General Orders and it was suggested by General Codrington, who had taken over on the death of Lord Raglan in 1855, that donations should take the form of a day's pay. Professor Smith refers to this as 'a compulsory levy on the troops'.[35] However, most of the covering letters suggest that the offerings were made without coercion, although, of course, the absence of such a letter may indicate perfunctory duty. In spite of some carping remarks about the Fund by army surgeons in the end the army contributed £9,000. Moreover, apart from official collections, there were a number of individual donations from soldiers and soldiers' widows, some of which were clearly heartfelt. One of the most poignant came from 'seven wounded soldiers who were discharged in Liverpool and who were nursed by Miss Nightingale'. Between them they collected 15s 6d and they asked that their names appear on the list. They are duly recorded in *The Times*. The coastguards, HM Dockyards and the Royal Navy all sent subscriptions, sometimes accompanied by personal letters and even poems.

It was the aim of the Fund Council to invoke all classes and to this end various people were approached and asked to take collecting books. The replies often have a familiar ring with recipients of the letters claiming that they were too obscure, too ill, burdened with work, or of the wrong political or religious persuasion to undertake such a task. One or two people said they thought that too much fuss was being made about Miss Nightingale and mentioned other 'heroines'. On the whole, in terms of cash, it is doubtful whether the collecting books were worth the time the secretaries expended in placating complaints of duplication and omission. In an age that believed in 'letting their lights so shine before men that they may see their good works' there were endless complaints about money not acknowledged and names misspelt on the subscription list, or worse still, not appearing at all.

The Fund was eventually wound up at the end of June 1856 when the total stood at £44,039. On 20 June, before the Fund closed, a Deed of Trust was drawn up between Miss Nightingale and the official Trustees. This indenture recites the resolutions leading to the appeal which raised £40,000 now invested in exchequer bills in the names of the Council members, Sir John Liddell KCB, MD having replaced the Earl of Ellesmere who had died. The composite resolution put to the meeting in November 1855 had stated that Miss Nightingale must have the power to direct the Fund; now clause 13 laid down that, for the purpose of enabling Miss Nightingale to exercise her powers with the latitude and freedom of action intended, the Trustees were bound to act in matters of investment, buying and selling under her direction. Clause 13 seems also to indicate the way Miss Nightingale was then thinking about a plan for nurse training:

> It shall be no means considered as obligatory... that land be purchased or a building erected... but buildings may be hired or the intended institution may be such as not to involve a special establishment in order to meet the objectives of the Fund.[36]

This suggests a training attached to a hospital rather than an independent school, college or Home which would serve as a Motherhouse on the continental pattern.

The Deed gave wide powers to Miss Nightingale, but the Council and Trustees were apparently happy that this should be so since, as she put it, 'the field was so new' and only she knew what she wanted and how to interpret pragmatic experience. As it happened, all too soon, greater delegation became necessary and a second Deed had to be drawn up.

The collecting of nearly £45,000 – possibly over £2,000,000 in today's money[37] – in 20 months says much for the diligence, ingenuity and sheer hard work on the part of the organisers. They were of course taking the current where it served, and advantage of the fact that the press had built Miss Nightingale into a popular heroine and the subject of sentimental ballads and broadsheets. It is also likely that many people, including some politicians, who had become horrified at the course the war had taken, were glad of some diversion and perhaps the one good thing to praise and come out of the whole sorry story.

The Nightingale Fund was probably the first national appeal aimed at all classes which in itself is a comment on the fact that under the impact of industrialisation the old class divisions were changing. Artisans now subscribed to 'causes'. Unfortunately the lists of subscribers are not necessarily accurate, there is some duplication and the various lists do not tally, but from the lists in *The Times* it is possible to get a broad picture of how the money was collected and from where it came.

Although the appeal was aimed at all classes it seems to have been largely an aristocratic and upper-class affair. The bulk of the money came from generous individual donations, the highest being £300, but with a good sprinkling of £25 and over from the upper middle class and the upper echelons of the Church. The minor aristocracy and the well connected were well represented and there were often several subscriptions from within the same family. Interestingly enough, and perhaps shedding light on women's property rights and the numbers of unmarried women, there was a large number of women subscribers where the sums were not so large but for whom Miss Nightingale must have had a special significance. Finally there was the blessing of the Court. Queen Victoria felt strongly about the army and what Lady Longford describes as 'her own magical balance on the point of the military pyramid'.[38] Queen Victoria admired Miss Nightingale, and like Miss Nightingale the Queen felt there was a special bond between her and the army. The approval of the Queen was reflected in the donations of those around her.

Perhaps the importance of the appeal, however, was not so much the £45,000 it garnered, but that it focused the minds of people, especially intelligent middle-class groups, on the fact that nursing was a suitable occupation for respectable educated women and that nurses needed to be trained.

Notes

1. *The Times*, 'Despatches from the Crimea', 9, 12 and 13 October 1854.
2. Woodham-Smith, C., *Florence Nightingale* (Constable, London, 1860), p.135.
3. Verney, H. (ed.), *Florence Nightingale at Harley Street* (J.M. Dent & Sons, London, 1970).
4. Cook, Sir E., *The Life of Florence Nightingale* (Macmillan, London, 1913), p.199.
5. Stanmore, A., *Sidney Herbert – A Memoir* (Murray, London, 1906), vol. 1, p. 401. (Stanmore is undoubtedly biased in favour of Sidney Herbert and he thinks Miss Nightingale hectored and exaggerated and could only see good in her own circle.)
6. Cook, *Florence Nightingale* , vol. 1, p. 258.
7. Woodham-Smith, *Florence Nightingale*, p.196.
8. Depuy, T.N., *Encyclopaedia of Military History* (Macdonald, London, 1970), p. 990.
9. Cook, *Florence Nightingale*, vol. 1, p. 262.
10. Sidney Herbert as reported at the Manchester meeting, GLRO, HI/ST/NC18/21, 17 January 1856.
11. Cook, *Florence Nightingale*, vol. 1, p. 141.
12. Cope, Z., *Florence Nightingale and the Doctors* (Museum, London, 1956), p. 20.
13. Cook, *Florence Nightingale*, vol. 1. p. 269, FN to S. Herbert, 27 September 1855.
14. S. Herbert to S.C. Hall, August 1855, GLRO, A/NFC/29/1.
15. S.C. Hall to B. Bolt, 5 November 1855, GLRO, A/NFC/36/6.
16. Minutes of the NFC, GLRO, A/NFC/27/1, 8 November 1855.
17. Report of the proceedings of a public meeting held in London, 29 November 1855, GLRO, HI/ST/NTS/36/1.

18. GLRO, A/NFC/27/1, 20 December 1855.
19. FN to S. Herbert, *Herbert Papers*, Wilton House, vol. 1856, 6 January 1856.
20. Ibid., vol. 1859, 25 May 1859.
21. Nightingale, F., *Subsidiary Notes as to the Introduction of Female Nursing into Military Hospitals in War and Peace* (Harrison & Sons, London, 1858), pp. 1–9.
22. FN to Selina Bracebridge, *Herbert Papers*, Wilton House, vol. 1856, February 1856.
23. Smith, F.B. *Florence Nightingale – Reputation and Power* (Croom Helm, London & Canberra, 1982), p.73.
24. Cook, *Florence Nightingale*, vol. 1, p.272.
25. GLRO, A/NFC/29i, 6 January 1856.
26. S. Herbert to Md. Goldschmidt, GLRO, A/NFC/27/1, 20 March 1856.
27. S. Herbert to S.C. Hall, GLRO, A/NFC/29/1/52, 22 January 1856.
28. Ibid.,/27, 23 January 1856.
29. Ibid.,/39, 6 January 1856.
30. Ibid.,/21, 25 November 1856.
31. S. Herbert to FN, BL, Add Mss 43394, 22 March 1856.
32. (Illeg.) to S. Herbert, GLRO, A/NFC/29/1/36, April 1856.
33. Covering letter with n. 19 (above), *Herbert Papers* Wilton House, vol. 1856.
34. Lefroy-Baker to SH, GLRO, A/NFC/29/1, May 1856.
35. Smith, *Florence Nightingale*, p. 156.
36. Deed of Trust Clause 13, GLRO, A/NFC/1, 20 June 1857.
37. *Sunday Telegraph*, 'Purchasing Power of the £ 1825–1980', compiled by Barry Bowyer (1982).
38. Longford, E., *Victoria, R.I.* (Pan Books, London, 1964), p. 308.

2. Founding the Nightingale School

Say not the struggle naught availeth,
The labour and the wounds are vain,
The enemy faints not, nor faileth,
And as things have been they remain.
…

In front the sun climbs slow, how slowly
But westward, look, the land is bright.

Arthur Hugh Clough, 1st Secretary to the Nightingale Fund Council

Miss Nightingale returned to England in July 1856, first to Embley then to Lea Hurst where she set about dealing with the accounts and claims arising from the Crimean war.[1] In August her old family friend, Sir James Clark, physician to the Queen, arranged for her to meet the Queen and the Prince Consort at Balmoral. Miss Nightingale accepted because her one overriding aim was to get an independent enquiry into the muddle and inefficiency of the Army Medical Service. She was accompanied to Scotland by her father and on the way stayed with Sir John McNeill at Birk Hall, who helped her to prepare her case. At the same time she took the opportunity of visiting hospitals in Edinburgh, visits that were later to give the Fund a number of contacts but a good deal of anxiety.

The meeting with Victoria and Albert was a success but there was no hope of action and a Commission unless the Palmerston administration agreed to an enquiry. In spite of the fact that the hectoring of *The Times*, the invective of Lord John Russell and the broadsheets from the Court about the mismanagement of the war had brought down the Aberdeen administration, Palmerston, on taking office, had ignored the report of the McNeill and Tulloch mission. The critical findings of this enquiry and of others – including that of the radical Roebuck – had been swept under the carpet by the convenient Chelsea

20

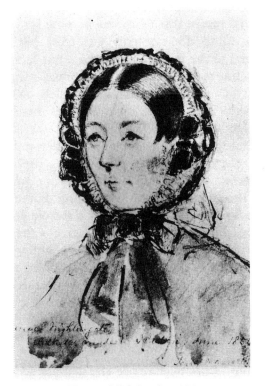

Florence Nightingale, 1856

Board.[2] Once home Miss Nightingale, who knew the facts, was determined to use her influence to right this wrong. Her first task was to persuade Lord Panmure, now Secretary for War, to set up a Royal Commission and, as Panmure was noted for never doing today what could be put off until tomorrow, persuasion took much time and energy.

In November 1856 Miss Nightingale moved into the Burlington Hotel in order to be on hand for the fray, and as Panmure dilly-dallied she threatened to play her ace and publish her own report.[3] Fortunately in the spring of 1857 the possibility of an expeditionary force to China concentrated the minds of the War Office wonderfully and, with Panmure's reluctant blessing, a Royal Commission started to function in May. It was during this period, while she was agitating for the Commission, that Miss Nightingale met Sir John Liddell, Director General of the Navy Medical department, who asked for her help in introducing female nurses into the naval hospitals. Miss Nightingale inspected Haslar Hospital and other naval establishments and this accounts for Sir John becoming a member of the Fund Council and for the subsequent interest of the Fund in the nursing at Haslar.

All this activity meant that there was no time for consideration of the Nightingale Fund, for not only was Miss Nightingale herself deeply committed to the Royal Commission, but so too were at least three leading members of the Council. The summer was taken up with the preparation of evidence; Miss Nightingale's own report, *Notes Affecting the Health and Efficiency and Hospital Administration of the British Army*, ran into 830 octavo pages. At the same time Miss Nightingale was waging a campaign to get the new military hospital at Netley built on the most modern pavilion plan like the Lariboisière Hospital in Paris.[4] A Christmas visit to her neighbour, Lord Palmerston, at Broadlands brought her support, but the elaborate new building on the Southampton waterfront on the old corridor style was far too advanced for the War Office to agree – the cajoling of the Prime Minister notwithstanding. Now Miss Nightingale spent much time and effort trying to suggest ways of overcoming the basic defects in construction, lighting and ventilation. It was in this connection that Lord Panmure asked Miss Nightingale to write a second volume of 'Notes'. These are generally known as *Subsidiary Notes – The Introduction of Female Nursing into Military Hospitals in Peace and War*.[5]

In these 'Notes' Miss Nightingale clarified her general ideas about nursing, for example, 'what it is, and what it is not', how it should be organised, how the ward tasks should be allocated, who would make the best recruits for this 'coarse, repulsive, servile, noble work' and how nurses should be paid.

Many of the ideas contained in these 'Notes' were to be put into practice in the Nightingale School which accounts for the military terminology much loved by Miss Nightingale and which has always been used in connection with nursing. Mrs Wardroper wrote in the register 'has left the Service' and 'absent on sick leave' and nurses were 'on duty' and, more rarely, 'off duty' with many of the ideas on discipline relate to the needs of military hospitals (see Chapter 6).

As well as writing these reports single-handed except for the help her cousin by marriage, Arthur Hugh Clough, now gave her, Miss Nightingale spent the summer visiting hospitals and concerning herself with hospital construction. The various articles she wrote in papers like *The Builder* eventually appeared as *Notes on Hospitals*,[6] a booklet which was to revolutionise hospital building, and in which she was helped by a member of the Fund Council, Sir Joshua Jebb, the Surveyor General of prisons who was the architect of the model Pentonville prison. Another influence on the 'Notes' was Edwin Chadwick, the Sanitary reformer, with whom Miss Nightingale corresponded. These streams combined to produce that 'model hygienic' institution that was so to typify the latter part of the nineteenth century.

At this stage little thought had been given to the use of the Nightingale Fund and Miss Nightingale herself had shown little interest in it or in nursing. Then in August 1857, while living and working at the Burlington Hotel in London, known to the campaigners for reforms in the Army as 'the little War Office', and coping with volumes of statistics and bullying Lord Panmure about the Royal Commission, she suffered a sudden collapse. Her symptoms included tachycardia, dyspnoea, insomnia, acute nausea and revulsion at the sight of food, all of which were attributed by her medical advisers to overwork. The received medical wisdom at the time was that it was unnatural for a woman to engage in excessive mental activity: it would surely lead to 'a nervous collapse'. The way to deal with the situation was to order complete rest and, of course, the cessation of all mental work. Other victims of this chauvinistic attitude include Charlotte Brontë, Harriet Martineau and Elizabeth Barratt, all of whom continued with mental effort and creative writing from their beds.

It is ironic that in 1857 bed rest was the only therapy available to doctors and Miss Nightingale obeyed. For this she has invited 140 years of speculation and much wasted ink by her biographers as to the cause of her illness. These include Cook, who shelters behind dilatation of the heart and 'neurasthenia' which was a blanket Victorian term for unexplained psychosomatic symptoms.[7] Cope believed it was stress induced by her struggle with officialdom.[8] Pickering attributed it to an anxiety neurosis brought about by her unresolved conflict with her mother and sister.[9] Smith inferred it was downright malingering in the pursuit of power.[10] To these can be added more recent suggestions. In the great debate on myalgic encephalomyelitis Florence Nightingale has been recruited as an example of the 'misunderstood sufferer'. Other suggestions have been lead poisoning due to her childhood being in the vicinity of mines and, even more bizarre, the suggestion of syphilis. None of these explanations is convincing. Neurasthenia is meaningless, and if the stress neurosis was due to her conflict with the War Office why did it continue for 20 years after the strife was over? Pickering's argument is attractive but it does not explain why the symptoms continued after Parthe had married in 1858 and she was 'henceforth left alone'; moreover, the conflict with the family has been greatly exaggerated.[11] The 'ME' theory is hardly consistent with the patient's ability for continued and almost Herculean work.

It seems strange that these eminent physicians who were called to this patient, who was now a national figure, did not consider her past history. While in the Crimea in 1855 she had a severe attack of 'fever' from which it was thought she would die; she eventually emerged so emaciated, agitated and depressed that she was hardly recognised. What was Crimean Fever? There have been many suggestions including typhoid and typhus. Florence Nightingale herself claimed it was typhus.[12] The third possibility was 'Remittent Fever' sometimes known as 'Malta' or 'Mediterranean' fever caused by *Brucella melitensis*, and this as Dr Young[13] has shown was the most likely culprit for Florence Nightingale's attack in 1855 and for much of her subsequent illness. It is a fever that if it becomes chronic produces serious complications and often a personality change, and can be indistinguishable from neurosis.

Although Miss Nightingale herself has left us some colourful descriptions of what she was to call her 'Thorn in the Flesh' – 'T in the F' to her correspondents – including her spinal pain, nausea and insomnia, few of her biographers have charted the course of her illness as Dr Young has done, but if we look at this, it explains much about her attitude to the Nightingale Fund. In 1859, while negotiations with St Thomas's were underway, she had a second and severe attack with cardiac symptoms, nausea and muscular weakness; both she and her doctors thought she would die, and her obituary was brought up to date. She wrote 'last letters', was sorry to 'leave the nursing scheme in the lurch' and suggested that Mrs Shaw Stewart was the only person fit to take over. One senses that this was the least of her worries.

The symptoms subsided although she was still plagued by insomnia, headaches and depression. In 1861, after the Nightingale School had been started, she had another and this time more severe attack with new symptoms including spinal pain, paraparesis when she was unable to walk, dyspnoea due to chest spasms and depression which was no doubt exacerbated by the deaths of Sidney Herbert and Arthur Clough; again she wanted to die: 'This is the shortest day, were it my last'.[14] She now became bed or couch ridden for the next six years, during which time she continued to work on the Indian Report, the Army Medical Service, the Poor Law reform and the design of hospitals. Then, towards the end of the decade, she had a remission and it is at this stage that she took an interest in what was happening at St Thomas's; she was not happy with what she found. By the 1870s most of her symptoms had disappeared and after 1880 the depression lifted and she resumed something like normal relations with her family and friends, a change that is manifest in her letters. Is it possible that she was a burnt-out case?

Like other Victorian invalids it is impossible to separate the clinical symptoms from the iatrogenic effect of the treatment: the year of 'bed rest', the social isolation, only seeing one person at a time, the opium needles and the laudanum to ease the pain. Although irritability and depression are part of the constellation of Brucellosis sequelae, there must have been a psychosomatic underlay, and there is no doubt that with her capacity for dramatisation Florence Nightingale used her illness to get work done: being at death's door concentrates minds wonderfully. She used her friends and relations mercilessly, at times making accusations that were intemperate so that it is small wonder that less sympathetic biographers have labelled her a liar. Was this change of personality due to bouts of fever and pain? In her youth she had been affectionate and given to sentimental friendships, but like so many thoughtful adolescents she had been given to periods of depression and self-doubt interspersed with periods of euphoria. Did her illness merely exaggerate these tendencies, or was it, as Dr Young suggests, a change brought about by her Crimean Fever? This we will never know. But even her detractors will admit that whatever means she used 'for the sake of the work' the result justified them.

Although the Fund was provided to found a training for hospital nurses it is by no means sure that this would have been Miss Nightingale's priority. In 1860 she wrote to Sir John McNeill:

> Missionary nurses – these are our aim. Hospitals are an intermediate stage of civilization. While devoting my life to hospital work I have come to the conclusion that hospitals are not the best place for the poor sick except for surgical cases.[15]

In *Notes on Hospitals*, when referring to the mortality rate in city hospitals, she writes:

> Facts such as these have sometimes raised doubts that in all probability the poor sufferer would have had a better chance of recovery at home... a vast deal of the suffering in these establishments is [from] avoidable causes.[16]

Miss Nightingale increasingly believed, and rightly so, that proper sanitation, ventilation and the right food would banish much current sickness. Writing to Dr Pattison Walker in 1866 she said that the purpose of medicine should be to 'make the public care for its own health'.

For this reason she saw nursing as more than a mere handicraft but rather as a sanitary mission. In a curious way, and by the same reasoning, Miss Nightingale was blindly and fanatically against the germ theory of infection. 'There are no specific diseases', she reiterated, even when men like Koch had demonstrated that there were. This attitude coloured her views on nurse training and made her fearful that the new scientific training and lectures from medical men like Bernays at St Thomas's would turn nurses into 'medical women' and deflect them from their proper task of being sanitary missioners. In a letter to Edwin Chadwick, who agreed with her views, she wrote: 'Sanitary science has so disproved the invisible, seminal contagions that I can only see a mania for being wrong in such letters as Greenhow's and Simon's.'[17]

Therefore, apart from more pressing concerns like the evidence to the Royal Commission, the collection of statistics, the health problems of India and the Poor Law reform, Miss Nightingale was still ambivalent about how hospital nursing should, or could, be developed. This uncertainty is important because it is reflected in Miss Nightingale's changing attitudes to nursing as a 'profession' and who should be selected as nurses, what their tasks should be and, above all, how they should be prepared to meet those tasks. The fears about nurses becoming imbued with ideas about bacteria made her suspicious of doctors' lectures and what was later to be described as 'the medical model'. Her fears in this respect were often justified – but for the wrong reason. However, she was soon to find out that if 'tradesmen's and farmers' daughters' were to be trained even in the handicraft of nursing they needed educated women to teach them. Furthermore, educated women were necessary to teach the public 'to care for its own health'. Miss Nightingale's difficulty was that she had no body of nursing knowledge or educational theories in order to substitute 'nursing matters' for medical knowledge, and the educated women brought in to teach the less educated all too soon absorbed medical knowledge.

In November 1857, three months after the onset of her illness, Miss Nightingale wrote to her uncle, Samuel Smith, who was managing her affairs, 'I have thought about what you said, that I ought to make a will about *that* money' (the Nightingale Fund), and, showing a certain amount of indifference, she continues:

> I think it would be much better left to the Council. I know no one but Mrs Shaw Stewart who would be any good (or anything but harm) with the money – and I know she would not take it. I really believe that the way to do the best would be to leave it to St Thomas's where the R.M.O. and the matron have ideas of raising the nurses but can't because the treasurer won't give the funds... Please advise me.[18]

This was 1857 and Miss Nightingale was in communication with Mr Whitfield at St Thomas's about Mrs Shaw Stewart doing a private training, and Mrs Shaw Stewart had written about Mr Whitfield's ideas.

Three weeks later Miss Nightingale wrote in a similar vein to Sidney Herbert saying that she was sorry to leave the nursing scheme in the lurch and recommended Mrs Shaw Stewart. At this stage, at the end of 1857, she clearly had not given any serious thought as to how the money should be used and was not, it seems, very interested.

Although Miss Nightingale was considered to be at 'death's door' her epistolary output was undiminished. During this time besides sanitary problems she returned to her metaphysical work *Suggestions for Thought* which she had begun in 1852.

In considering Florence Nightingale's attitude to health care and nursing it is important to look at her own spirituality and her tortuous path through conflict and doubt. Her parents, influenced by the philosophies of the Enlightenment, were liberal in outlook and were both Unitarian. However, when they inherited property and with it squirearchial duties they became members of the Church of England and the girls were brought up in its tenets. Through her parents, as a young woman, Florence met scholars from Europe, some educated in Germany where they had imbibed the philosophies of Schopenhauer and Engels and the new Biblical criticism. One of these was Chevalier Bunsen, ambassador to the Court of St James 1842–54, a theologian and scholar of ancient and oriental languages who had a great influence on the young Florence. Another influence was Julius von Mohl, married to Mary Clarke. It was through the Bunsen circle that Florence met Richard Monckton Milnes. At this stage she was out of sympathy with the Church of England, which was trying to come to terms with the 'new criticism', with the Tractarians at odds with the Evangelicals and both torn by doubts arising from archaeological evidence and new historical interpretation and translations.

At the same time Florence, an impressionable young woman, was attracted to mysticism. At the age of 17 years she received what she thought was a 'call from God', though in later life she doubted whether anyone heard the voice of God telling them what common sense would not have told them.[19] She studied the lives of mystics like St Teresa of Avila and in 1848, while in Rome, took instruction from Madre Sta Columba in the Convent of Trinita De Monte on how to accept the will of God. For a time she was attracted to the Church of Rome and later, in 1853, she actually wrote to Henry Manning, who had recently converted to Rome, asking for advice on conversion. Not surprisingly Manning, who had read her *Suggestions for Thought*, thought that her views were too radical.

Meanwhile, with her amazing capacity for learning she had become interested in the theories of Adolphe Quetelet, the Belgian statistician, who believed that human behaviour, including criminal behaviour, could be found in antecedent and coexistent conditions[20] and, if these were corrected, human behaviour could be changed. Florence

Nightingale took Quetelet's theories and applied them to health. If the conditions that caused ill health could be changed, mankind would become healthy and there would be no need for nurses for the sick, only nurses to promote health. It was for this reason that she was implacably opposed to the germ theory of infection: it deflected people from 'sanitary science' which was the foundation of good health.

Having rejected the literal interpretation of the Bible, miracles and the efficacy of prayer – do not pray to be delivered from cholera, just clean out the gutters and supply clean water and a proper sewage system – she argued that there is a reason for everything; it is up to mankind to find the reason.

It was these different, if sometimes contradictory, influences that led her to attempt *Suggestions for Thought*. She thought that the Artizans of England were being led into atheism by Positivism and the doctrines of Auguste Comte, who argued that all knowledge must be based on verifiable fact. She therefore set out, at the age of 32 years, to give the working class a philosophy that would accommodate their doubts, yet guide them to a spiritual dimension, which she described as a Universal Law and God's Law, God's Law being manifest in Nature which was unalterable.

The exegesis, set out in three volumes and printed privately, is confusing, prolix, often repetitious, and the general effect is chilling. In its composition Florence Nightingale was no doubt influenced by Arthur Clough, who, like a number of Victorian intellectuals, had lost his faith and his university post and who was now living at South Street, 'tying up parcels for Miss Nightingale'.

In 1859 he sent the manuscript to Benjamin Jowett, his old tutor at Balliol, for consideration. Jowett himself was a radical thinker and had been involved in the current controversy over the new translation of the Bible. Although he dismissed the work as being 'too full of antagonism' he recognised 'the inprint of a new mind' and later became her guide, philosopher and friend, eventually steering her back into what became known as 'the Broad Church' which accommodated such radical thinkers as men like Dennison Maurice, the founder of the Christian Socialist movement, with whom Miss Nightingale corresponded and had some sympathy.

It is only by understanding Florence Nightingale's concept of social engineering and her religious philosophy that we can understand her attitude to health and nursing. In *Notes on Nursing* she says that it is the nurse's duty to put the patient in a position for Nature to act on him, Nature being God's Law; the nurse must assist that law by providing the right conditions, that is by fulfilling the sanitary mission. This is why we get the misused quote 'the less knowledge of medicine that matron had the better, it does not improve her sanitary practice. [21]

In *Notes on Nursing* Florence Nightingale argues that only when we have done away with the pain and suffering that are due not to disease, but to the absence of the conditions that are necessary for Nature's reparative process, will we know what are the symptoms of the suffering that are inseparable from the disease. Rob van der Peet argues that Florence Nightingale saw the suffering accompanying disease as a moral or religious, rather than a sanitary, issue and that she favours a theological rather than a medical notion of disease.[22]

This leads to the hope expressed in *Suggestions for Thought*:

> The history of human nature is the history of progress towards feelings and manifestations that we distinguish as MORAL right or righteousness. God's Law is such that the history of man is tending to bring about such feelings in human nature.[23]

The nineteenth-century feeling of optimism in the possibilities of science and the improvement in human nature characterises 'The Whig Interpretation of History'.[24] Florence Nightingale was not alone in this philosophy.

Besides being a sanitary missioner the nurse must be a role model and a good influence, hence the insistence on 'you cannot be a good nurse without being a good woman'. This is why Miss Nightingale always insisted that the training of the character in a nurse was as important as the acquisition of knowledge.

Suspected of Socianism because of her Unitarian background, an admirer of Roman Catholic nuns, with friends among High Anglicans and with heretical views on the Bible, perhaps explains why the Evangelical Agnes Jones had written to her in 1865: 'How is it that no one denies your philanthropy but everyone doubts your Christianity?' to which she had replied that she was indeed 'A poor follower of Christ'.[25]

For Florence Nightingale the test of religion was to live it. For this reason the Nightingale School was open to all creeds, or none; she judged people not by their adherence to a particular sect or creed but by their moral character and integrity.

The Army Medical College which opened in 1860 at Fort Pitt at Chatham arose out of one of the recommendations to the Royal Commission, namely, 'to institute an Army Medical School', the purpose of which was to provide postgraduate training for doctors entering the Army Medical Service. The course, she insisted, must be two years – much longer than the army thought necessary – the entrance must be by competitive examination and the final passing out and ultimate posting should be partly determined by examination results. This is particularly interesting in the light of Miss Nightingale's later comments on the fact that examinations for nurses were of little value. The other interesting comparison was Miss Nightingale's insistence, against all-comers, that the Army Medical School should be independent with tutors selected purely for their teaching ability, and not because they had held positions in the army or were well-known consultants. Moreover Miss Nightingale was against the doctors paying fees for their course because they had already paid for their medical training and she thought that the army itself should foot the bill.

No doubt part of the difference in Miss Nightingale's attitude to what was necessary for nurse education arose from purely pragmatic considerations: the need for medical education was already established, the need for nurse training was not, and it would be necessary to proceed slowly and experimentally. However, there was a more fundamental reason: Miss Nightingale saw the main object of nurse training as being the development of character and of self-discipline with moral training being more important than mere academic education. The distinction between the qualities necessary for medical practice and for nursing was made succinctly by Henry Bonham Carter in 1882[26] but it was a distinction hard to explain and often not understood by even the most distinguished of the Nightingale acolytes.

In February 1858 the Palmerston administration fell and Lord Derby formed a government with Sidney Herbert, now Secretary of State for War and the Colonies. At last Herbert had the chance to push for the reforms he had been planning and, once again, everything conspired against time being given to the Nightingale Fund. In March of that year Miss Nightingale wrote to Mr Herbert pleading illness and asking to be relieved of the responsibility for 'the large Fund which is called by my name which was so generously placed in my hands...'[27] This provoked an immediate reply telling her that she had been 'too curt' and to think again. Dutifully she replied on 27 March, hardly enthusiastically, but saying 'I will work if I can when I can... but the fear of neglecting the trust committed weighs heavily.'[28] It can hardly have escaped Mr Herbert's notice that Miss Nightingale was working like a slave on subjects that interested her more, including the rebuilding of St Thomas's.

As Miss Nightingale made this plea, Mr Herbert, no doubt in consultation with Mr Bowman who was co-founder of the Nursing Sisters Order of St John, made the suggestion that the Fund should use King's College Hospital and make arrangements with the St John's sisterhood. The idea had merit. The superintendent, Mary Jones, was Miss Nightingale's 'dearest friend' whose correspondence with Miss

Nightingale helps to fill the lacunae in the story of the early Nightingale school, and later she and Mr Bowman made visits to St Thomas's and advised on the nursing programme. Mr Herbert was no doubt favourable because of the association with the late Charles Blomfield who as Bishop of London had led the Church reform movement fostered by Peel.[29]

It was a suggestion with which Miss Nightingale, ill though she said she was, did not concur. Six sisters from St John's had gone with her to Scutari and four had returned home because they would not accept her discipline; probably more importantly, Miss Nightingale knew from experience with Miss Stanley's 'Puseyites', who came out to the Crimea independently, what havoc Lady ecclesiastics could wreak. Miss Nightingale may not have been too certain about the form nurse training should take, but one thing she was sure about was that the Fund, collected as it was from all denominations, must avoid the *odium theologicum*.

Before her illness Miss Nightingale looked at London hospitals and possible superintendents and there is a letter from Mrs Shaw Stewart saying, 'I have spent a month in this fine hospital [the London] but it would be useless for you to undertake the matronship unless you are prepared to spend several years there.'[30] Mrs Shaw Stewart had known Miss Nightingale well in the Crimea and this may have been a perspicacious remark. She knew that Miss Nightingale had no intention of being a superintendent. The Middlesex was considered as was the University College Hospital, and another possibility for the Fund was the Royal Free. Mr Carter Hall, the joint secretary to the collecting committee, clearly favoured this solution and sent a letter and a good deal of literature about the Royal Free and its advantages to Miss Nightingale.[31] Miss Nightingale thanked Mr Hall but there is no indication that she entertained the suggestion seriously.

Miss Nightingale herself says that during the spring of 1859 she was in contact with many hospital authorities. During February and March she corresponded with her old friend Dr Elizabeth Blackwell, whom she had known since 1850, in the hope of persuading her to be the superintendent. However, Miss Blackwell wished to practise as a doctor, a choice Miss Nightingale deprecated, but Dr Blackwell eventually – and wilfully – returned to America.

If all the correspondence during the spring of 1859 is taken into account and read in its proper sequence, there is some justification for thinking that the much-quoted letter of 24 May, in which Miss Nightingale finally tells Mr Herbert that St Thomas's is the only place,[32] is to some extent a rationalisation of a decision already taken for other reasons.

Miss Nightingale had been writing to Mr Whitfield, the Resident

Medical Officer of St Thomas's Hospital since 1856 when she was in Balaclava. Mr Whitfield supplemented his income by taking nursing students and in 1856 Miss Nightingale wrote to Mr Whitfield thanking him for Mrs Roberts and commending Mrs Shaw Stewart, who had been the superintendent at Balaclava and was keen on being a surgical nurse rather than a superintendent, saying that 'Mrs Shaw Stewart will give any remuneration agreed on.'[33]

Mr Whitfield was an apothecary and in spite of his now enhanced position would have been considered a parvenu by his medical colleagues. He continued the correspondence and presumably enjoyed his new relationship with the Nightingale circle. In 1856 he sent Miss Nightingale his booklet, *The Administration of Medical Relief to Outpatients at Hospitals*.[34] The pamphlet sets out the Chadwickian view that it is false economy on the part of Poor Law authorities to skimp medical care and he quotes the Bence Jones report on the St Pancras Infirmary, a philosophy he thought would appeal to Miss Nightingale.

By 1858 Miss Nightingale had become well known for her articles in *The Builder* on the construction of hospitals[35] – a subject in which Mr Whitfield now had a vested interest. As long ago as 1832 the medical staff of St Thomas's were complaining that the hospital was 'decayed and dilapidated' and were advocating rebuilding. In the meantime the situation had been exacerbated not only by the decline in the neighbourhood and the crumbling of buildings but also because of the close proximity of Guy's Medical School which was taking more and more students.[36] Suddenly, in 1858, the South Eastern Railway Company gave notice of their intention of taking part of St Thomas's garden in order to extend the line from London Bridge to Charing Cross. Opinion was divided as to whether to compel the Railway Company to buy the whole site, or to retain some of the land and rebuild in Southwark. Most of the Court of Governors were in favour of getting the railway to take all the land and rebuilding elsewhere.[37] Mr Whitfield, influenced by Miss Nightingale, and men like Farr and Chadwick who were currently writing on the subject, was in favour of moving to the suburbs and he solicited Miss Nightingale's support.

There now begins a close correspondence. In November 1858 Miss Nightingale was responding to an offer by Mr Whitfield to look at the sanitary arrangements in Edinburgh for her and she asks him:

> Please get the statistics of the mortality of nurses such as you were kind enough to send me from St Thomas's. I have all the London hospital statistics which I will whisper to you privately – 54 per cent of the deaths of nurses are preventable.[38]

These were presumably the figures that were given her by Dr Farr and which she published in *Notes on Hospitals*.[39]

Mr Whitfield had two main problems: first, to get the Railway Company to buy all the land and to pay well for it; and second, to get enough votes for a move into the suburbs. On both counts Miss Nightingale was a valuable ally. To achieve the first she asked Sir James Clark to influence the Prince Consort, who was one of the governors, and at the same time she persuaded her brother-in-law, Sir Harry Verney, and other friends who were Members of Parliament to lobby support for an injunction in Chancery to restrain the Railway Company from taking possession of the garden without purchasing the whole site, a tactic which was to prove successful. To obtain the second objective, which was more difficult, Miss Nightingale and Mr Whitfield planned a campaign to win public opinion. Mr Whitfield collected the admission tickets of accidents which showed that St Thomas's was already serving the suburbs, and these he showed to Miss Nightingale who released them to *The Builder* which had already published a number of her articles. An unsigned article now claimed there was an opportunity for the public to get a double benefit: 'An extension of a railway system and to rebuild a noble charity in a dry, healthy suburban area.'[40]

There was a flurry of correspondence between Miss Nightingale and Mr Whitfield with 21 letters in February and March alone. On 19 February Mr Whitfield wrote that he favoured removal to a healthy location and the building of a model civil hospital, to which Miss Nightingale replied: 'You have the opportunity to build the finest hospital in the world if you do but take advantage of it.' She suggested Blackheath with offices and casualty at Southwark and transporting the patients by railway: 'Treat the London sick like the war wounded.'[41]

The doctors, led by Mr Flint South, the senior surgeon, did not see it that way and were furious at the publication of the figures which they considered as being used to draw spurious conclusions. On 19 March an article in *The Lancet* disagreed with *The Builder* and insisted that St Thomas's Hospital must remain in 'A populous district for those seized by sickness or maimed by accident.' The next week *The Builder* riposted using more statistics to prove the point and Miss Nightingale got *The Times* to take a supporting line. However, three years later in 1862, John Simon, then Superintendent General for Health at the Privy Council (to whom the Whitfield–Nightingale School of thought was an anathema[42]), in his campaign to keep St Thomas's in the heart of London to serve its poor, got *The Times* to take a different line and Delane became a supporter of the Lambeth site.[43]

At this stage, March 1859, there is a significant letter from Mr Whitfield, which says:

> If you are well enough and could spare the time I should like to have some conversation with you most particularly on the subject you mentioned to me last Saturday, the inability you felt from the state of your health personally to superintend the appropriation of your fund for nurses.[44]

The following weeks saw much lobbying by both factions; Mr Whitfield wrote that he was 'canvassing support among the doctors and Sir Charles Barry had agreed to the plan of Lariboisière'.[45] From other correspondence it is clear that Mr Whitfield was seeing Miss Nightingale and they were discussing plans for a Nursing School at St Thomas's; presumably without consulting the Council, she had laid certain plans before him because only four days after the letter quoted above there is a letter from Mr Whitfield which says:

> The class of women who now supply the hospitals with sisters and nurses could or would not undertake a hundredth part of what you wish to impress upon them as essential, they are too bigoted to their habits and customs to entertain the philosophy of it... it would be impossible to find women capable of undertaking the competitive examination you have drawn out.[46]

Considering Miss Nightingale's later views on examinations the last sentence is amazing. It is unfortunate that we have not got the draft plan that she put to Mr Whitfield so that we can see how far she modified her views and bowed to his argument.

During this period we have Miss Nightingale's word that she was corresponding with Dr Blackwell whom she hoped would be the superintendent of the School, but in March Mr Whitfield warned her that Dr Blackwell would *not* be acceptable at St Thomas's.[47]

At the beginning of April Miss Nightingale saw Sir John McNeill and must have put him to the tentative plan for an arrangement with St Thomas's Hospital. The following day he wrote:

> It would seem as if you had one choice supposing St Thomas's accept your proposal, of either beginning there, or waiting until you have *trained some suitable matron for some other hospital*... I would venture to add I would not sacrifice any object affecting the ultimate success for the sake of having something done a year sooner... You propose to make nursing a respectable profession and to give it the public security of a certificate... must not all who gain certificates be left to pursue their profession in the manner and in the field that may be most advantageous to themselves...[48]

This then is the background of the letter sent by Miss Nightingale to Mr Herbert on 24 May, in which she says:

> I have discussed the matter with some of the authorities at St Thomas's. The Matron of that hospital is the only one of any existing hospital I would recommend to form a School for nurses. It is not the *best conceivable* way of beginning. But it seems to me the *best possible*. It will be a beginning in a very humble way. But at all events it will not be beginning with a failure, i.e. the possibility of upsetting a large hospital – for she is a *tried* matron.[49]

In other words the explanation of that final sentence was that she had given in to St Thomas's – and Mr Whitfield in particular – on the subject of the superintendent because they had insisted on using *their* matron as part of the price of the deal.

Parsons, in his *History of St. Thomas's Hospital*, says it is interesting that Miss Nightingale chose St Thomas's when 'the medical school was in low water, the staff rather difficult and [there was] probable disorganisation'.[50] Apart from the fact that Miss Nightingale regarded medical students as a corrupting influence and their absence a blessing, and that she was confident that her advice would prevail and that St Thomas's would arise like a phoenix as the most modern hospital in the world – in the suburbs – there were other reasons. It seems as if Miss Nightingale was caught in the web of her own Machiavellian intrigue to get St Thomas's rebuilt to her plan, and in accepting Whitfield's *quid pro quo* she had made certain concessions. First, she had accepted his recommendation for a superintendent. At this stage, as far as we know, she had only seen Mrs Wardroper twice. Second, Mr Whitfield had poured cold water on her original plan for nurse training and she had modified it. Presumably, it was at his instigation that the 'contract to give service', clause 6, was inserted. Could it be that Mr Whitfield and the hospital authorities had an interest in the future service needs of St Thomas's Hospital?

Mr Whitfield's attitude to nurse training is interesting because he was chosen by the Fund Council to be the main instructor of the probationers and was paid for his services, yet as early as 1863 he was writing that he did not approve of the 'Combination of diaries [nursing] with case taking... and the introduction of points of nursing into the history of case and medical treatment, I think would be objectionable.' By the time of the great schism in 1872 Mr Whitfield's views on nurse training make those of Mr South and his oft quoted comparison with housemaids look almost advanced.

In retrospect it looks as if Miss Nightingale in her anxiety to achieve one objective, better hospital construction, sacrificed a scheme for

nurse training to expediency. Sir John McNeill, displaying characteristic Scottish caution, obviously did not approve. Standing Voltaire on
his head he was saying that the good and the expedient would be the
enemy of the best. Moreover, he seemed to doubt that the proposed
plan would raise nursing to a profession, because to the nineteenth-
century mind the quintessential professional man was independent of
contracts and charged his own fees. Charles Bracebridge was to
express the same doubts and it is significant that Sir John McNeill did
not attend a meeting of the Council once the agreement with
St Thomas's was drawn up.

In May, Sidney Herbert, who was now Minister of War and busy
with other matters, and whose plan for King's College Hospital had
been overruled, acquiesced in the St Thomas's scheme. The main
concern of the active members of the Council was how to make it a
workable undertaking. Sir John McNeill wrote to point out that the
Council as now constituted was inefficient and there must be an executive committee of people in London who could exercise power and a
paid secretary.[51] Sir John suggested Arthur Clough, a cousin by
marriage of Miss Nightingale, who was a scholar and who, after
throwing up his fellowship at Oriel, became principal of University
Hall in London and was subsequently an examiner in the Education
Office.[52] Clough was also a poet of distinction who had abandoned his
academic career because of religious doubts and had been helping
Miss Nightingale to whom he was devoted. Strachey describes him
somewhat unkindly as ending his career 'tying up brown paper parcels
for Miss Nightingale'.[53] Miss Nightingale was unhappy about the
suggestion because Clough was a relative, but it was pointed out that
he was the only suitable person and he would be a servant of the
Council. Clough, hesitatingly, eventually accepted:

> I will serve as long as Miss Nightingale gives guidance, afterwards the
> cause would be a different one. She spoke of the following questions
> requiring consideration:
>
> 1. If the whole of the establishment of nurses be not put under the
>   direction of the Nightingale Council, will not the authorities defend
>   their nurses against ours? their nurses will be jealous of ours who are
>   to take their place.
> 2. How are women to know about the advantages offered at the hospi-
>   tal – how are they to be advertised?[54]

From this it is clear that no firm plan had been drawn up and that
Miss Nightingale was contemplating taking over all the nurses at
St Thomas's.

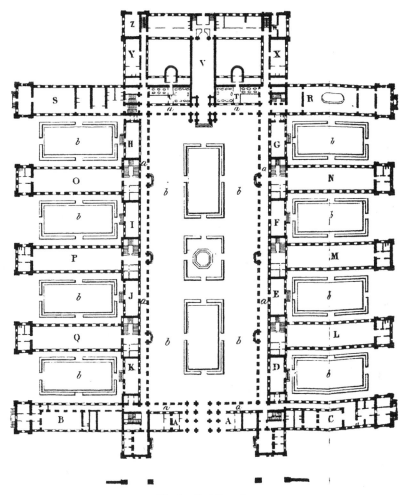

The Lariboisière plan

During the summer negotiations between the Railway Company at St Thomas's Hospital continued with the Company paying £296,000 for the whole site. Mr Whitfield visited new hospitals including the much favoured Lariboisière in Paris and reported their merits to Miss Nightingale. The arrangements for the training school seem subsidiary to the interest in rebuilding and, such as they were, they seem only to have been discussed by Miss Nightingale, Mr Whitfield and Mr Baggallay, the Treasurer, and there seems no record of Miss Nightingale seeing Mrs Wardroper until 1860 when she wrote to Sir John McNeill, 'I must see the matron.'

On 19 December Sidney Herbert summoned the first meeting of the Nightingale Fund Council to the War Office. In a letter to Sir John McNeill the week before, he had written: 'I grieve to say that she [Miss

Nightingale] is failing badly but to have this business settled will be a relief to her mind.'[55] A week previously a new Deed of Delegation[56] had been drawn up, and Miss Nightingale was now using her ill health to push the plan with St Thomas's as quickly as possible and to divest herself of responsibility. Now the Nightingale Fund Council had to endorse the Deed of Delegation and accept a scheme in which it had played little part.

At this stage Miss Nightingale sent a long and detailed scheme to Sir John McNeill suggesting how the Council should proceed:

> The present matron and nurses to continue to perform their duties and instruct pupil sisters and nurses who may enter until these are suffi-ciently numerous and competent to take charge of an entire ward.

The letter goes on to set out the accommodation to be agreed upon, attendance at lectures, hours of repose and the fact that the matron must be responsible for the strict observance of rules and that

> the matron keep a book to be called the discipline book in which shall be entered daily every instance of misconduct or act of omission calling for punishment or serious reprimand.

After setting out an elaborate scheme for gradually replacing the staff in the hospital by Fund trainees, taking half from the current staff and half from new entrants, the letter ends: 'the primary object to be the establishment of a normal school for nurses with a view to the elevation of that class to the position of a profession'.[57] This letter is interesting because the scheme eventually agreed between the Fund Council and St Thomas's Hospital is very different and there is little evidence that the existing staff at St Thomas's ever became trainees under the Fund or that the staff were ever replaced on a proportional basis. What actually happened in June 1860 was something very different from Miss Nightingale's outline in December 1859. Probably St Thomas's were not prepared to have their nurses ousted by what Professor Smith calls the 'cuckoo in the nest'.[58]

The Deed of Delegation stated that the Council was to appoint a committee of four with full powers. The named persons were Sir John McNeill, Sir James Clark, Mr William Bowman and Sir Joshua Jebb – three doctors, two of whom were elderly, and a prison reformer. Miss Nightingale also authorised the appointment of Arthur Clough as secretary at £100 a year, 'his generous offer of acting in an honorary capacity not being accepted'. The fact that the committee had full powers made the Nightingale Council largely redundant. This Council had been named by Miss Nightingale when she was in Scutari to give it respectability and assurance to the donors, but some members like the Dean of Hereford and Bence Jones were never to attend a Council meetings again.

The committee met in Mr Bowman's rooms on 7 March 1860 when it was agreed that negotiations be started with 'the President, Treasurer and the Governors of St Thomas's hospital and that they be requested to form a sub-committee to deal with the matter'. The following day Arthur Clough called on Richard Baggallay who Whitfield described as a 'very deep old fox' to make arrangements for a conference which was held with remarkable promptitude on 17 March.[59] The conference agreed that certain wards at St Thomas's could be used to give instructions to probationers under the Fund and that the matron should also be the Lady Superintendent under the Council of the Fund. On Miss Nightingale's insistence the matron was to have the power to select the probationers and to dismiss them; the matron should also recommend a number of sisters to give instruction to the probationers and a medical officer to give medical instruction. The Council, or the committee acting for it, had the power to appoint an instructor to give elementary knowledge in reading, writing and arithmetic. It was also agreed that a certain number of nurses at present employed were to be selected as probationers with a view to receiving instruction and gaining the Fund's certificate. It is impossible to be sure from the register but there is no evidence that this clause was implemented. The Fund agreed to pay the Court of Governors £22 a year for the board and lodging of each probationer, £100 a year to the matron, £50 a year to the medical officer to give instruction and £10 a year to the teaching sisters. These payments were of course over and above the salaries paid.[60] Mrs Wardroper was already receiving £150 a year, a house, board and lodging and a servant and must have been among the most highly paid women of her day. It has been calculated that Mr Whitfield from various sources was already getting £643 15s 10d average income exclusive of apprenticeship fees, together with his house and an allowance of coal; consultant physicians and surgeons at the time were receiving an average of £239 9s 0d and £488 3s 6d respectively.[61] Mr Whitfield was on the way to becoming a wealthy man.

The estimates by Baggallay and Clough on a scrap of paper show that they reckoned that 15 probationers would cost the Fund about £800 a year which they worked out in units of five as:

£110   for board and lodging
£ 60   for wages at £12 a year
£ 32   for washing and for use of the furniture.

£202

In addition the overheads would be

£100   for the matron
£ 50   for the medical officer
£ 50   for 5 sisters at £10 each.
—————
£200

Fifteen probationers would therefore cost £606 + £200 + administrative costs. Each probationer would on this reckoning cost the Fund £60 a year. This was by no means parsimonious on the part of the Fund since the average remuneration for a sister was £30 a year and if another £30 was added for the cost of board and uniform a probationer was costing the Fund as much as a sister was costing St Thomas's.

During subsequent committee meetings the draft agreement was discussed and corrected. Sir Joshua Jebb visited the hospital to make arrangements for providing separate lodgings for the probationers and further meetings with the governors resulted in the agreement being reduced from the proposed seven years to an experimental two years. The committee of the Fund had had second thoughts.

The final agreement was drawn up in May 1860.[62] Advertisements were placed in certain papers during the month and the Regulations for Training Probationers' Nurses were set out and signed in June by Arthur Clough. The wage was reduced to £10 but was offset by the offer of a gratuity of £3 or £5, according to the class of the award, on evidence of the nurse serving a year in hospital following the training. Subsequent agreements allowed for gratuities to be paid after each year in the three years succeeding the completed training when the nurse 'was required to enter into service as a hospital nurse in such situations as may from time to time be offered them by the committee'. While this agreement helps the historian to trace what happened to the early nurses, this form of contract was soon to be the source of much controversy.

There are several things to notice about the first agreement. First, an extra, quite generous payment is made to the sisters to give instruction, but no one seems to have vetted their ability to do this. Second, Mrs Wardroper was given absolute power although at this stage she had had little contact with the Nightingale Council. Third, applications from the present staff were anticipated in spite of Miss Nightingale's searing remarks about the standard of behaviour of the average hospital nurse. Fourth, it was a contract for the servant class. Candidates, if successful, were given some outdoor clothing, presumably to ensure that they looked respectable, a small wage, some of which was held back until there was evidence of good behaviour. Everything was 'found' including tea and sugar and a washing allowance because 'nurses ought to be compelled to have certain changes of linen weekly which they will not do if they are compelled to pay for themselves'.[63] Finally, there was the suggestion that there should be help with reading and writing which hardly anticipates the recruitment of educated women.

Moreover, although Miss Nightingale had drawn up her famous character sheet under 14 heads (see Appendix I), which was to be filled in monthly to ensure that the probationers were proficient in various nursing skills and gave satisfaction as to traits of character, there was no way of checking that such a return had any value. Although Mrs Wardroper visited the wards perhaps more than most matrons, she was not a nurse and did not pretend to be one. No one seems to have asked who would watch the watchers.

In view of the subsequent events a letter from Mr Bracebridge in June 1860 is worth quoting because it indicates that the Fund Council was not unanimous:

> I object to the regulations for nurses in the following particulars. It was always intended from the first and since to establish a profession, and to give incentive to those in it to rise by grade, grades only to be obtained by certificated experience and character, to be rewarded by hospital rank and the pay of private service. A nurse after twelve months should be free to take any service...

This part of the letter should be compared with the doubts expressed by Sir John McNeill; both seemed to sense that the contract scheme was exploitation and 'unprofessional'. Mr Bracebridge goes on:

> Further, Mrs Wardroper as superintendent. I object that she or her successor may commit acts of tyranny if she can expel without the leave of [a] sub-committee. This will also act against good women taking service and it would be a pleasanter thing for her to refer to a tribunal of appeal. Again the Register should be named that of the Nightingale Fund and not confused with the hospital.[64]

In an acerbic postscript Mr Bracebridge goes on to complain about the wording of the contract on pay and clothing which he says is such as 'effectively to exclude lady nurses'. Mr Bracebridge was more prophetic than he knew. It is worth comparing this letter with one that Mr Bonham Carter received from a Mr Carr concerning Miss Osburn's contract in 1867[65] and also Miss Nightingale's later confession that she had 'greatly altered her mind about the power given to the matron'.[66]

We can only conclude that the contract took the form that it did during the long and tortuous negotiations between Miss Nightingale and St Thomas's. In his letter to Miss Nightingale in March 1859 Mr Whitfield had made clear his low expectations for nurses and Mr South's views on nurses as housemaids were well known.[67] Was the lowering of expectations the price Miss Nightingale paid in order to get an agreement with St Thomas's? We shall never know because much of the bargaining took place in private.

On 9 July 1860 the first probationers arrived. There is no evidence as to how they were selected, which advertisements they answered, and how many were already hospital nurses. It seems that Caroline Stone, aged 22 years, was sent by the authorities in Bath since she returned there to be the matron, where she remained for many years. But wherever they came from the first intake was hardly encouraging. Four were quickly dismissed, two for disobedience, one for being drunk, one for ill health, while Charlotte Dixon died at the end of her training from typhus. Of the remainder, two had scarlet fever and another typhus but recovered; only four were still nursing and able to collect their promised gratuity at the end of the second year.

Miss Nightingale, who in 1861 was devastated by the deaths of Arthur Clough and Sidney Herbert, and overwhelmed by the pressure of work concerning the Indian Sanitary Commission, seems not to have noticed the events at St Thomas's. The committee members of the Fund and the Trustees, whatever their private misgivings, reported favourably in public. Mrs Carter Hall wrote an article in eulogistic style for the *St James's Magazine*[68] and the first report of the Council expressed 'quiet satisfaction'. Since during the first year's vacancies were filled in a haphazard manner and record keeping was not Mrs Wardroper's forte, it was possible to present the figures in a more favourable light. But however the figures are interpreted it was a 'a beginning in a humble way'.

Notes

1. GLRO, HI/ST/NC/8, 6 July 1856.
2. MacAlister, F., *Memoir of the Rt. Hon. Sir John McNeill*, quoted in Cook, Sir E., *The Life of Florence Nightingale*, vol. 1, p. 336.
3. FN to S. Herbert, *Herbert Papers*, Wilton House, vol. 1856.
4. *The Builder*, 'Sites and Constructions of Hospitals', August and September 1858.
5. Nightingale F., *Subsidiary Notes as to the Introduction of Female Nursing into Military Hospitals in War and Peace* (Harrison & Sons, London, 1858).
6. Nightingale F. *Notes on Hospitals*, 3rd edn (Longman, Roberts & Green,

London, 1863).

7. Cook, *The Life of Florence Nightingale*, vol. 1 (Macmillan, London, 1913), p. 49.

8. Cope, Z., *Florence Nightingale and the Doctors* (Museum, London, 1954).

9. Pickering, Sir G., *The Creative Malady* (Allen & Unwin, London, 1974).

10. Smith, F.B., *Florence Nightingale – Reputation and Power* (Croom Helm, London, 1988).

11. Baly, M.E., *'As Miss Nightingale Said...'* (Scutari, London, 1991), Chapter 2; Vicinus, M. and Nergaard, B., *'Ever Yours Florence Nightingale'* (Virago, London, 1989).

12. GLRO/HI/ST/NC 1/70/6 Florence Nightingale/Mrs Cox, 1 August 1870.

13. Young, D.A., Florence Nightingale's Fever. *British Medical Journal*, 23–30 December 1995.

14. Florence Nightingale/Mary Clarke, 21 December 1861. Copy from the Wellcome Institute.

15. FN to Sir J. McNeill, GLRO, HI/ST/NCI/SU132, 13 August 1860.

16. Nightingale F., *Notes on Hospitals* 3rd edn (Longmans, Roberts & Green, London, 1863). pp. 4 and 7.

17. Cope, Z., *Florence Nightingale and the Doctors* (Methuen, London, 1958). See also Lambert, R., *Sir John Simon 1816–1904* (MacGibbon and Kee, London, 1963), p. 267; FN to Sam Smith, BL, Add Mss 43398, 19 September 1858.

18. FN to Sam Smith, BL, Add Mss 45792, 6 November 1857, f. 68.

19. Nightingale, F., *Suggestions for Thought to the Searchers after Truth among the Artizans of England*, 3 vols (Eyre & Spottiswoode, London, 1860, printed privately).

20. Quetelet, A., Sur l'homme et la développement de ses faculties: physique sociale (1835). Quetelet was the founder of the Statistical Society of which Florence Nightingale became a member.

21. Cope, *Florence Nightingale and the Doctors*, p. 77.

22. Peet, R. van der, *The Nightingale Model of Nursing* (Campion Press, Edinburgh, 1995).

23. Nightingale, *Suggestions for Thought*, vol 3.

24. Butterfield, H., *The Whig Interpretation of History* (Pelican, London, 1973).

25. Baly, M.E., *'As Miss Nightingale Said...'* 2nd edn (Baillière Tindall, London, 1997), p. 29.

26. The case for the opposition to the RBNA petition, GLRO, HI/ST/NTS/A 17/1. See also H. Bonham Carter letter to *BMJ*, September 1879.

27. FN to S. Herbert, *Herbert Papers*, Wilton House, 23 March 1858.

28. Ibid., 27 March 1858.

29. S. Herbert to FN, BL, Add Mss 43394, 22 March 1858, f. 21. See also Chadwick, O., *The Victorian Church* (Adam & Charles Black, London, 1970), part 2, p. 365.

30. Shaw Stewart to FN, GLRO, HI/ST/NC2/v5 (illeg.), 1857.

31. S.C. Hall to FN, GLRO, A/NFC/62 (n.d.).

32. Woodham-Smith, C., *Florence Nightingale* (Constable, London, 1950), p. 344. See also *Herbert Papers*, May 1859.

33. FN to R.G. Whitfield, GLRO, HI/ST/NC3, SU181, February 1856.
34. GLRO, A/NFC/AC75/27. See also Hodgkinson, R., *Origins of the National Health Service* (Wellcome Historical Medical Press, London, 1967).
35. *The Builder*, 'Sites and Constructions of Hospitals' (1858), no. 99, p. 100.
36. Parsons, F.G., *History of St. Thomas's Hospital*, vol. 3, (Methuen, London, 1956), Chapter 2.
37. Papers relating to the dispute with the Charing Cross Railway Company, GLRO, HI/ST/NC1/58, 1–3.
38. FN to R.G. Whitfield, GLRO, HI/ST/NC1/58, 6a, November 1858.
39. Nightingale, *Notes on Hospitals*, Table 2, p. 4.
40. *The Builder*, 26 February 1859 (A/NFC/63/2).
41. FN to R.G. Whitfield, GLRO, HI/ST/NC1/59/1, 21 February 1859.
42. Lambert, *Sir John Simon*, p. 479.
43. *The Times*, March 12, 13, 17, 20 and 24 1863.
44. R.G. Whitfield to FN, GLRO, A/NFC/63/15, 14 March 1859.
45. R.G. Whitfield to FN, A/NFC/63/14, 11 March 1858.
46. R.G. Whitfield to FN, BL, Add Mss 47742, 18 March, 1859, f. 65.
47. Cope, *Florence Nightingale*, p. 145.
48. J. McNeill to FN, BL, Add Mss 45768, 11 April 1859, f. 94.
49. FN to SH, *Herbert Papers*, vol. 1859, 24 May 1859. See also Woodham-Smith, *Florence Nightingale*, p. 344.
50. Parsons, *St. Thomas's Hospital*, vol. 3, Ch. 2.
51. J. McNeill to FN, BL, Add Mss 45768, 11 April 1859, f. 94.
52. *Oxford Companion to English Literature*, 3rd edn (ed. Harvey) (Oxford University Press, London, 1946), p. 170.
53. Strachey L., *Eminent Victorians* (Chatto & Windus, London, 1918).
54. A. Clough to J. McNeill, GLRO, HI/ST/NC3/SUII, 26 April 1859.
55. S. Herbert to J. McNeill, GLRO, BL, Add Mss 45768, 15 December 1859, f. 106.
56. GLRO, A/NFC/2/1, 21 December 1859.
57. FN to J. McNeill, GLRO, HI/ST/NC3/SU123, December 1859.
58. Smith, F.B., *Florence Nightingale – Reputation and Power* (Croom Helm, London, 1982), pp. 158–9.
59. GLRO, HI/ST/NTS/AI/1, 17 March 1860.
60. GLRO, HI/ST/NTS/AI/3.
61. Prince, J., Unpublished thesis, 'The Nightingale Training School Reform of Nursing', p. 77.
62. GLRO, HI/ST/NTS/AI/3.
63. Nightingale, *Subsidiary Notes* (1954 edn), p. 44.
64. C. Bracebridge to A. Clough, GLRO, A/NFC/66, June 1860.
65. Carr to H. Bonham Carter, GLRO, HI/ST/NC18/17, 18 April 1967.
66. FN to H. Bonham Carter, BL, Add Mss 47719, April 1876, f. 23.
67. Woodham-Smith, *Florence Nightingale* , p. 345.
68. Hall, Mrs S.C., 'Something of What Florence Nightingale Has Done and Is Doing', *St James's Magazine*, vol. 1, April–July 1861.

3. St Thomas's Hospital Moves to Surrey Gardens

It is easy to potter and cobble about patients for a year without knowing the reason of what is done, so as to be able to train others.

Florence Nightingale

Within 18 months of the signing of the agreement with St Thomas's Hospital untimely death deprived the Nightingale Fund of both its chairman and secretary, a blow which left its eponym inconsolable, more prone to ill health and, for the time being, largely uninterested in the Fund.

By the spring of 1860 Sidney Herbert was already terminally ill with kidney disease; in December he was created Lord Herbert of Lea that he might give up his work in the Commons for the less arduous life of the Lords. He worked to the last and died at Wilton on 2 August 1861, aged 51 years old. Meanwhile Arthur Clough, always frail, grew worse and was ordered abroad, dying in Florence on 12 November, only 42 years old. After a brilliant start at Oxford Arthur Clough had been plagued with religious doubts and later he had become devoted Miss Nightingale, his cousin by marriage, being content, as he put it, 'to do plain work for his moral good'.[1]

The Fund Council meeting in July 1861, with both its chairman and secretary dying, had also accepted the resignation of Sir James Clark because of his ill health. At Miss Nightingale's request three new members were appointed: Mr John Forbes Clark, Sir James's son, a barrister who also married into the Nightingale family and who served the Council until his death in 1910; Mr William Spottiswoode, the Queen's printer, who had been a friend of the Nightingale family; and Sir Harry Verney, Member of Parliament for Bucks, and Miss Nightingale's brother-in-law who became the chairman of the Council and remained so until just before his death at the age of 93 years. At the same time Miss Nightingale prevailed upon her cousin, Henry

Bonham Carter, a barrister aged 34 years, to stand in for Clough. Young Mr Bonham Carter wrote the minutes that July day and continued to do so for the next 53 years. Henry eventually gave up his work at the bar and took a salaried post as managing director of the Guardian Fire Insurance, the Fund becoming his life's work with the management committee consisting of Nightingale relatives or close friends. Like the Renaissance Popes, Miss Nightingale felt safer with her family and old friends. It is from Miss Nightingale's correspondence with her cousin Harry that much of the day-to-day business of the Fund can be reconstructed because, unlike Arthur Clough, Bonham Carter only saw Miss Nightingale when he considered it necessary, saying tactfully, that he did not want 'to tire her with a visit for what could be done by letter'.

While Miss Nightingale nursed her grief and prepared to do battle for Lord Herbert's unfinished reforms, St Thomas's Hospital prepared to move to a temporary home. After much delay and a letter from the Prince Consort who advocated a 'more healthy locality in the suburbs'[2] the Railway Company had taken all the land. While the governors decided on a new site and the hospital was built, a much reduced St Thomas's was housed in what were once pleasure gardens with a music hall and a zoo in Newington.

The Fund Council considered moving the Nightingale School to Guy's or King's College, but rather than risk disruption, Mr Bonham Carter thought it safer to stay with St Thomas's.[3] However, in view of the fact that there were only 200 beds at Newington and the accommodation was limited, it was recommended that the number of probationers be reduced to ten.[4] Sir Joshua Jebb, who was chairman until his unexpected death in 1868, inspected the accommodation and was insistent that there was a bedroom for each probationer. In actual fact in the next year Mrs Wardroper took 13 probationers, but as the two Miss Merryweathers came for only two months as observers and five candidates were rapidly dismissed – one for 'alcoholism and drug taking' and one for 'indiscretion towards students' – the accommodation problem presumably resolved itself. In 1864 the intake was increased because Mr Rathbone paid for extra accommodation in order that nurses could be trained for Liverpool (see Chapter 5).

In 1862 a new agreement between the Fund and the probationers[5] provided that the Fund should give a year's training to the successful candidate at the end of which, if they were satisfactory, their names would be placed on a 'register' which would contain a record of their conduct and qualifications. At the end of their year probationers were now expected to 'enter into the service as hospital nurses in such situations as may be offered them by the Committee for the next 5 years'. In 1872 this was modified to three years, and in any event, as Miss Nightingale was later to point out, the contract could not be enforced. The Fund dropped the idea of awarding 'first and second class certificates' and gratuities were now paid for satisfactory service for three years after training.

What the probationer would be expected to do and to learn was set out on the back of the application form from 1861–71 as follows:

DUTIES OF PROBATIONER

You are required to be sober, honest, trustful, trustworthy, punctual, quiet and orderly, cleanly and neat.
You are expected to become skilful –

1. In the dressing of blisters, burns, sores, wounds, and in applying fomentations, poultices, and minor dressings.
2. In the application of leeches, externally and internally.
3. In the administration of enemas for men and women.
4. In the management of trusses, and appliances in uterine complaints.
5. In the best method of friction to the body and extremities.
6. In the management of helpless patients, i.e. moving, changing, personal cleanliness of, feeding, keeping warm, (or cool,) preventing and dressing of bed-sores, managing position of, &c.
7. In bandaging, making bandages, and rollers, lining of splints, &c.
8. In making the beds of the patients, and removal of sheets whilst the patient is in bed.
9. You are required to attend at operations.
10. To be competent to make gruel, arrowroot, egg flip, puddings, drinks for the sick, &c.
11. To understand ventilation, or keeping the ward fresh by night as well as by day; you are to be careful that great cleanliness is observed in all the utensils those used for the secretions as well as those required for cooking.
12. To make strict observation of the sick in the following particulars:–

The state of secretions, expectoration, pulse, skin, appetite; intelligence, as delirium or stupor; breathing, sleep, state of wounds, eruptions, formation of matter, effect of diet, or of stimulants, and of medicines, &c.

13. And to learn the management of convalescents.

Timetable for the Probationers under the 'Nightingale Fund' (1862)

DAY

Rise	Breakfast	Wards	Dinner	Wards	Exercise	Tea	Wards	Dormitory	Supper	Bed
6 a.m.	6½ a.m.	7 a.m.	1 p.m.	2 p.m.	3½ to 5p.m.	5 p.m.	6 p.m.	8½ p.m.	9 p.m.	10 p.m.

NIGHT

Rise	Tea	Wards	Dormitory	Breakfast	Wards	Dormitory	Exercise	Dinner	Bed
9 p.m.	9½ p.m.	10 p.m.	6 a.m.	6½ a.m.	7 a.m.	10 a.m.	11 a.m. to 1 p.m.	1 p.m.	2 p.m.

During the week prayers are read in the wards at 8 a.m., and in the Dormitory at ¼ before 10 p.m. On Sunday the Probationers are expected to attend Divine Service in the Parish Church at 11 a.m.

BY ORDER

By 1862 the Fund were already allocating part of their income of £1,426 8s 6d to midwifery training and they now calculated they were spending £1,071 a year on the training at St Thomas's which meant each probationer was costing £70.[6] University College Hospital, which already had a training system with the Sisters of All Saints, applied to the Fund for help, but reluctantly the Council had to reply that 'now it had no means available'.

As the battle for the suburban site for St Thomas's continued in the medical press and *The Times*, Miss Nightingale herself appears to have been more interested in the new St Thomas's than what was happening in Surrey Gardens. She did, however, express herself disappointed in the candidates, and said that she did not blame Mrs Wardroper but rather 'the lack of publicity due to the uncertainty hanging over the future of St Thomas's'.[7] It was therefore agreed that the chairman, Sir Joshua Jebb, should give a 'Statement of the Appropriation of the Nightingale Fund' to a meeting of the Social Science Association. This was a useful way of making the work of funds or charities better known as the reports were printed and could have a wide circulation.

The Statement gives a lucid, if expurgated, account of the history of the Fund. Sir Joshua stressed that the objects of the Fund was

> to afford the means of acquiring a thoroughly practical and scientific training to woman desirous of becoming nurses... hospital nurses were chosen because it was the object most prominently put forward by the subscribers, and properly so... it is to hospital infirmaries that those patients resort who are in most need of assistance... it is on the efficiency of nurses in hospitals more than in any other position, that a larger number of cases are dependent for successful treatment.

There follows a glowing outline of the arrangements with St Thomas's, the regulations for admission, the terms of training and the fact that moral training was as important as the scientific aspect and, therefore, 'only those who are impressed with a strong sense of duty in desiring to improve themselves and do a credit to their calling are admitted'. Sir Joshua admitted there had been some difficulty in finding such candidates:

> Persons of superior manners and education, ladies in fact are not as a rule required, but rather women of somewhat more ordinary intelligence belonging to classes in which women are habitually employed in earning their own livelihood.

In this Sir Joshua was faithfully reflecting Miss Nightingale's view about the women who made the best nurses, but he continued, leaving himself a loophole:

> Ladies are not excluded, on the contrary where sufficient evidence is shown that they intend to pursue the calling as a business, and have the qualifications that will fit them to be superintendents their admission would be considered an advantage.[8]

As publicity the Statement was superb, but there was a certain elliptical regard for the truth. By stressing the importance of hospital training in voluntary institutions Sir Joshua disregarded the fact that such hospitals only provided 11,000 beds[9] and most of the sick were in their own homes, in Poor Law institutions and even in his own model prisons and such patients were more dependent on nursing because there was little medical cover. Second, the claim that the training was scientific was spurious, lectures were few, there was no co-ordination of theory and practice, there had been no evaluation of the so-called trainers as persons able to educate others, and, as was soon to be discovered, there was no way of knowing whether assessment had any value. Last, by suggesting that ladies would be welcome to prepare themselves on the same course as ordinary probationers as a training for superintendence, Sir Joshua touched on a dilemma that the Fund never resolved. It was a dilemma inherited by twentieth-century nursing and which it never resolved. If there were to be two types of entry for two different positions when 'trained', should there not be two types of training?

The result of this publicity and other various magazines articles was that the secretary to the Fund and Miss Nightingale herself were inundated with letters from hospitals and institutions asking the Fund to supply them with trained nurses. All the letters were dutifully answered; unfortunately we do not have all Henry Bonham Carter's replies, but the difficult were referred to Miss Nightingale, for whom, on occasion Dr Sutherland sometimes replied as in the case where a shipowner wanted a trained nurse for sick mariners: 'tell him to make his ships fit for human beings then his mariners would not require nursing of any kind'.[10] What Henry Bonham Carter replied does not survive. However, as time went by Henry developed a distinct style of his own and there seems to have been less referral.

Perhaps up to half of the some 2,000 letters in the Bonham Carter collection are concerned with requests for, or advice about, staff. The replies were polite but firm. Because it represents the requirements and the philosophy of the Fund a reply to Lord Beauchamp is worth quoting. The Fund had received a letter which stated that Worcester had an excellent matron ('the daughter of a clergyman of some standing'), the nurses had separate bedrooms and comfortable quarters and they were paid £23 a year and there was ample domestic help. Worcester sounded a paragon, but Lord Beauchamp received this reply:

> The matron must be trained otherwise she is responsible for the conduct of the nurses and for placing them to the House surgeon and the nurses will have a surgeon for their master. The whole female staff ought to be responsible to the matron otherwise there is a lack of moral discipline... The matron will see that the nurses carry out the orders of the medical men in everything concerning the treatment of the patients: a complaint against nurses by medical men or patients should be made to the matron who alone should take action. Any complaint against the matron should be made to the committee.[11]

In a final coda which would be re-echoed by nurses in the next century, only less succinctly:

> Doctors are very liable to imagine that because they are the proper people, and the only persons, to give orders respecting the treatment of patients, therefore they must have the entire control of staff.

Time and again replies reiterated three main points. First, there could be no help from the Fund without a trained matron to whom the nurses were accountable for nursing matters. Second, the governors or committee must pay reasonable rates – £20 a year at least, with comfortable board and lodgings. In 1858 Guy's, which was considered fairly good, was paying £18 and full board.[12] Third, there must be adequate domestic help: nurses must not be scrubbers'.[13] For some the price was too high and vested interest over the first point too strong, but there were a few who made improvements and who acted as a grain of mustard seed. The Fund's influence in the early years was not confined to sending out missionary nurses, of which they had few to send, but it had a wider role as an advisory body.

In the meantime, by 1864, the 'Build in the Suburbs' faction at St Thomas's had lost the battle. John Simon, now a powerful influence, who rightly rejected as unproven the assertion that 'well conducted hospitals in towns were necessarily more dangerous to the health of their inmates than those outside'[14] ran what Royston Lambert describes as a brilliant campaign as an *éminence grise*. He persuaded the doctors and the governors that St Thomas's must remain in the heart of London and he personally negotiated with the President of the Board of Trade to ensure that the governors were offered the Albert Embankment site at a favourable rate. The governors were won over and accepted. Miss Nightingale was furious and never forgave Simon and wrote to the treasurer, Mr Baggallay, that 'The position is the worst in London and two feet above the water marker. Dr Leeson's proposal to warm with hot water should not be entertained.'[15]

She wrote in a similar vein to Sir John McNeill, who agreed. Once again Miss Nightingale and the anti-germ party had advocated the right thing for the wrong reason as was proved by the various reports on the sanitation of St Thomas's in the next 20 years. Moreover, had the plan to build in the suburbs been accepted there would have been one less teaching hospital within a five-mile radius of Westminster to plague the administrators of the National Health Service.

The architect of the new hospital was John Currey, the third of the Currey dynasty at St Thomas's and, although he designed the hospital on the Lariboisière pavilion plan, critics, including Miss Nightingale, thought that the blocks were too close.[16] The new treasurer at St Thomas's was Francis Hicks and there are now a number of hints suggesting a worsening relationship between the Fund and the Court of Governors. In 1865 it was necessary for the Fund Council to draw up a new agreement with St Thomas's Hospital. Sir Harry Verney wrote: 'I dislike binding ourselves to St Thomas's for longer than can be avoided – if is must be 7 years we must be cautious.'[17]

The Fund Council in general disliked the new site; the one reason for choosing St Thomas's was the expectation that it would be rebuilt in a more healthy situation. Moreover, the Council was now unhappy about the proposals for the probationers' quarters – what the Council called 'The Nurses' Home'. Miss Nightingale wrote that the architects and the governors did not seem to understand that

> ward training is but half of training. The other half consists in women being trained in habits of order, cleanliness, regularity and moral discipline... the whole establishment must be so constructed that the probationer's dining rooms and day rooms, dormitories and the matron's residence and office must be put together and the probationers under the matron's immediate hourly direct inspection and control.[18]

There are a large number of letters between the Fund Council and the hospital authorities on the proposed accommodation which was to put the probationers' sleeping quarters in the attics and the dining-rooms in the basement. The controversy raged round two issues that were interlinked: first, how many probationers could be trained, and second, the size, arrangement and situation of the accommodation that was to be provided by St Thomas's Hospital. Mr Bonham Carter was wary about letting St Thomas's provide too much accommodation:[19] first, the authorities would expect a long-term contract, and second, the Fund could not finance more than ten probationers. Miss Nightingale, on the other hand, thought the criterion should be the number who could be trained:

> the required accommodation should be limited by the number who can be properly employed about the patients – not by our friend [the

treasurer] because I am sure that we will come ultimately to train for people paying.[20]

This would seem to indicate that the idea of 'Special' paying probationers came from Miss Nightingale. However, the treasurer, having realised the value of probationers for staffing St Thomas's, encouraged the idea of expanding the school and Mr Whitfield, backed by Mrs Wardroper, suggested that up to 45 probationers could be trained by having two on each ward.[21]

The hospital plans were circulated to the Fund committee members who were invited to attend a meeting with the governors and those who could not attend were asked for comments. Sir John McNeill Clark was particularly colourful on the problem of the distance between the attic and the basement:

> Women need to repair to their bedrooms more often than men and stairs are not conducive to female health or morality... there is a need for women to have a proper sitting room with cushions, flowers etc.[22]

The problem about stairs and corridors was a real one; later, in connection with Netley, Miss Nightingale herself mentioned stories she had heard from the probationers about their being molested by porters and other people hanging around the stairs of St Thomas's.

A conference took place between the officers of the Fund Council and the Court of Governors on 30 November 1865, the outcome of which is known as the 1866 Agreement.[23] In this the governors agreed to accommodate 38 probationers according to the plans submitted and the furniture and furnishings to be agreed 'by mutual arrangement'. The provisions for the training of probationers and for their board and lodging were to continue as before. This was a blow to Mr Bonham Carter who had argued that, because of the advantages the probationers brought, the maintenance charge ought to be reduced or abolished.[24] The Fund further agreed to make the same payment to the officers who helped with training and 'not to allow the arrangements with other hospitals or training institutions other than the agreement with St. John's to interfere with the arrangements'. Reluctantly the Fund agreed to the contract being for seven years which Sir Harry described as a 'hard bargain' and the Fund was not able to carry the point about being consulted in the future if there were changes in the post of matron or the Resident Medical Officer, or changes in the status of those posts. It was because of the Fund's dissatisfaction with the agreement that Mr Whitfield suggested that the Fund 'get their own men on the Court of Governors to upset the clique behind R.B.'[25] ('R.B.' was presumably Richard Baggallay.)

The committee considered this and Sir John Clark suggested putting forward William Spottiswoode: 'a man for everything – imposing and has £12,000 a year'.[26] But at that time the idea does not seem to have been pressed. Nevertheless the committee were clearly unhappy about the outcome and as Sir Harry put it: 'they were dealing with a Fund collected in peculiar circumstances and they needed to be cautious, they had to convince the public that they were doing the best with the money'.

Miss Nightingale was very displeased. She did not like the agreement and the fact that they could not control the appointment of the matron or the RMO:

> What grounds have we to trust St Thomas's in the selection of another matron – they are the last persons we should trust – everything is won at the point of a sword. There may be trained some matron and staff of our own which we might take, e.g. the Middlesex Hospital – and Mrs Wardroper may train a matron at St Thomas's in the event of her death or retirement.[27]

Nor was Miss Nightingale alone in feeling that the Fund was being used by St Thomas's. There was a critical article in the *Pall Mall Magazine* and this was taken up by *The Lancet*:

> The Hospital takes the Fund's money and pays it out in douceurs – a quarter of the whole amount expended on training. Other hospitals would think themselves fortunate in having the gratuitous services of probationers without expecting to be paid for training nurses.[28]

With the fall of the Whig government in June 1866 and the advent of Disraeli, Miss Nightingale found she had less opportunity for influencing official activity at the War Office and she was able to give more attention to the Fund, and from 1868 the number of letters on the subject begin to increase. In 1867 Miss Nightingale had clearly begun considering alternative arrangements for the use of the Fund and was toying with the idea of an independent school:

> ... if we would get sufficient suitable probationers I should think the proper use of the Nightingale Fund would be to spend capital and interest in bringing up such probationers under Mr Whitfield and Mrs Wardroper – such probationers ought to perpetuate *our* school, not St Thomas's.[29]

Unfortunately, when she probed into what was happening the more disillusioned she became with the two people 'who are the only reason why we are at St Thomas's', and that idea fell through.

At the Committee meeting in February 1867 it was agreed that the

Fund could only support ten probationers and it was resolved that payment for board should, in certain cases, be required and where possible the cost of the board and salary should be obtained from the institution sending the probationer for training.[30]

There were now a number of reasons why the Fund considered advertising for what it called a 'Special' category of probationer. From the outset there had been resistance to the contract and it could not be enforced. The Merryweathers had only been 'observers', Miss Lees's mother had objected to her being 'staff' and Miss Rappe from Sweden and several others had not signed, and recently Mr Carr had advised his client, Miss Osburn, that this was 'not a contract that a lady could sign'.[31]

The Fund, however, had more pressing problems than the social niceties of contracts. The midwifery experiment at King's College was about to come to an end[32] but even so the entire income of the Fund could only support 18 probationers and this meant no experiments elsewhere. If the Fund was to supply St Thomas's with 38 probationers the only way to make ends meet was to charge those who could afford to pay, or the institution that sent them. To the criticism that paying probationers would not train under the same conditions as the ordinary probationers Miss Nightingale said it was like educating 'the lady with her cook', but that the ladies would rise to the position of superintendent, not because they were ladies but because they were educated. The inducement for doing this rigorous training under the same conditions was that they would earn four times as much in the end. When the idea of ladies doing training was attacked in the press she wrote:

> The aim is to make nursing an art. The first question (for an art) is not whether a person is a 'lady', a person working for her bread, or a person of the lower middle class. I do not see what this galimatias about 'ladies', volunteers etc. has to do with it. Is a lady less of a lady because she has trained herself to such a point that she can command the highest pay?[33]

Miss Nightingale saw nursing as an art to be acquired by practice and discipline – a training of moral fibre – not a mere gathering of technical expertise. From this standpoint it made sense to educate the lady with her cook and nursing clung to the common portal of entry for the next 70 years. The problem arose when the lady and her cook coped with the more abstruse lectures on chemistry together; the educated were treated like medical students and the uneducated floundered.

However, urgent though money was, it was not the only reason for the 'Special' category, because some Specials were 'free'. Often these were daughters of clergymen or educated women left in impecunious

circumstances who Mr Bonham Carter thought had leadership qualities; indeed some of the most successful came into this category
including Maria Machin and Rachel Williams. Regulations were
drawn up setting out the terms for 'Training of Special Probationers
in the Practice of Hospital Nursing.'[34] These stated that:

> the Committee were offering opportunities for gentlewomen to qualify
> themselves in the practice of hospital nursing on payment only of the
> cost of their maintenance. Only those candidates will be admitted who
> may desire eventually to become qualified for superior situations in
> hospitals and infirmaries.

The regulations go on to state that

> occasional vacancies will occur for the admission of gentlewomen free
> from expense together, in some cases, with a small salary during train-
> ing.

The paying probationers paid £30 a year in two instalments. In
spite of the many protests about the contract this was retained;
however a few years later it was recognised that there were women
who, because of anticipated family commitments, could not honestly
sign the contract and these were exempted by paying £52 a year – in
other words they brought themselves out of their indenture.

By the mid-1870s there were five types of probationers: the 'ordinary' who received a salary of £10 a year, the 'Free Specials' who had
no salary, the 'Free Specials' who received a small salary and the
'Specials' who paid £30 a year for their board and lodging. All these
signed the contract stating that for the next four years (after 1872 the
next three years) 'they would take employment in a public hospital or
wherever offered them by the Committee'. Finally, there were the
'Specials' who paid £52 a year and did not sign the contract. No one
paid for their training as is commonly supposed. That the Fund was
able to get young women to do this rigorous training, pay for their
keep and sign a contract says much for the paucity of job opportunities for women in the 1870s. As John Stuart Mill said, 'occupations,
law and usage made accessible to them are comparatively few that the
field of their employment is overcrowded'.[35] The gainers were, of
course, St Thomas's who received the same monies from the Fund but
who now had 38 probationers working on the wards without any cost
to the hospital.

It is not always easy to be sure which probationers came into which
category but according to the 1872 report 29 ordinary probationers
were admitted during the previous year and six Specials, according to
the accounts contributing £152. This did not make a great difference

but as the Fund did not have to pay the salaries of the Specials it meant that they were maintaining 35 probationers for £1,213 6s 6d and were still within their income.[36]

Back in Surrey Gardens training went on under considerable difficulties. The 12 or so probationers were housed in 22 Manor Place, about which Mrs Wardroper was frequently writing to Mr Bonham Carter. Rebecca Strong, aged 23, a deserted wife, who trained in 1867, has left an account of *Life in Surrey Gardens as I knew it in the mid sixties of the last century*.[37] This document is undated but it was presumably written in the twentieth century, probably some 40 or 50 years later, and the picture drawn may be affected by the benefit of hindsight and a general desire to show how things had improved. It is worth noting, also, that in late life Mrs Strong was in the opposite camp to Miss Nightingale, Mrs Strong having started a Preliminary Training School in Glasgow. The reminiscence is important, however, because we have few records from probationers themselves for this decade, and Mrs Strong highlights one of the reasons why hospital nursing had not developed at this stage – 'there was little nursing for the nurses to do'.

She describes the great Glass House divided into two floors then subdivided into wards by partitions eight feet high. 'Therefore,' she says ominously, 'you can imagine the noise'. The balconies were used for sanitary purposes where conditions were primitive and on the ground floor the ward kitchen was also the operating theatre, 'the mere mention of which I think is sufficient'.

At that time, the taking of temperatures and pulses and the testing of urine were the work of medical students and 'there being no records to keep not much was expected of the nurse'. The consultants inspected the wounds, the nurses made the poultices and the dressers dressed. Mrs Strong, Sir Joshua and other Council members who visited seem to have viewed the nurses' quarters from a different perspective. According to Mrs Strong there was no sitting-room and the dining-room was used for the occasional class; probationers worked from 8.00 a.m. to 8.00 p.m. with two hours off in the afternoon, seven days a week. Uniform was worn on and off duty, and consisted of an apron tied round the middle and, when off duty, a bonnet and shawl. Mrs Strong's recollections may throw a shaft of light on Mrs Wardroper who visited the wards 'occasionally by night as well as by day'. She goes on to say that Mrs Wardroper's end was a tragedy: 'going to meet the steamer on which her only child, a married daughter was returning, she met not the daughter but her coffin. No wonder she lost her grip on her work... ' However, Mrs Strong's recollection is at fault because Mrs Wardroper had four children; in 1868 one of her sons was doing fair copying for her and the Fund was paying him a grant.[38] Nevertheless there must have been some basis for thinking that Mrs Wardroper 'lost her grip' and it presumably applies to the time she was matron and before 1887.

Contrary to Miss Rappe and other 'recollections', Mrs Strong says that Mr Whitfield took an interest in the pupils[39] and this may have been true during the early years. He certainly wrote extensive 'General Directions for the Training of Probationer Nurses Taking Notes on Medical and Surgical Cases in Hospitals'.[40] These start with the encouraging information, 'as many patients die within 24 hours after admission to hospital it is important that the preliminary account should be made as soon as possible'. The Directions go on to state what should be recorded. Apart from factual information and the constitutional character and habits of the patient, there should be a concise and general history of the disease, how, and with what symptoms, it appeared... Describe the general appearance, countenance, state of pulse, skin, tongue, excretions particularly the bowel and the bladder.' There are four pages of detailed instructions including the finer points of auscultation and percussion: small wonder that when Miss Nightingale saw this paper she said, 'This is a medical student's paper rather than a nurse's.'

The special points she wanted engraphed were those outlined in the register as the particular *nursing* skills that the probationer was supposed to possess at the end of the year.[41] From the ensuing correspondence it would seem that Mr Whitfield did not understand the difference between nursing and medical histories, a confusion in which he was not alone, then or since. At this point Mr Whitfield seems to have lost interest for he decided that the combination of diary keeping and case-note taking was impossible and beyond the mental powers of probationers who only needed simple instruction. 'As regards the introduction of points of nursing into the history of the case I think it would be objectionable.'[42] But this of course is what nurse training was meant to be about, dovetailing the nursing procedures with the symptoms of disease. Although Miss Nightingale was unclear about how to obtain her objective, she alone seems to have had in mind a 'nursing model'.

The following year Mr Whitfield had his own troubles. Mr Adams, one of the governors, instigated an enquiry as to why Mr Whitfield had received 942 gallons of porter and 36 tons of coal during the past year for his house in Newington.[43] Mr Whitfield seems to have been caught up in the payment methods of his day. In 1857 it had been recommended that perks and fees be replaced by a salary 'except for free porter and coal'. Presumably Mr Whitfield was making up for any gap in the fees on the coal and porter. At the enquiry Mr Whitfield was supported by a testimony from Miss Nightingale, and the governors decided that he was too able and experienced to lose.[44] However, the Committee recommended the appointment of a medical superintendent and this was virtually a vote of censure. This proposed change of status was presumably the reason for the Fund Council wishing to be consulted about changes in the post of RMO. In the event the resolution was not put into practice but Mr Whitfield knew that he would not be the Resident Medical Officer at the new hospital and this may well account for his behaviour in the next few years. There is an indignant letter from Mrs Wardroper who declared that 'she was shocked and disgusted at the attack on Mr Whitfield,'[45] which is a pointer to their close working relationship. Several times Mr Whitfield wrote 'Mrs Wardroper and I think as one'. Mrs Wardroper was apparently a conscientious but unimaginative woman – Selina Bracebridge described her as 'uneducated' – who was probably overawed by the forceful character of Richard Whitfield, known for exercising his charm on women of all ages. Moreover, letters indicate that during this period both Mr Whitfield and Mrs Wardroper were frequently ill, and if Mrs Strong's account of the conditions in Surrey Gardens is anything to go by this is hardly surprising. During their illnesses they appear to have deputised for one another in matters relating to the Fund and it is hard to believe that Mrs Wardroper did not know of Mr Whitfield's 'little weaknesses'.

If Mr Whitfield and Mrs Wardroper were occasionally ill so too were the probationers. An accurate analysis of what happened to the early Nightingale nurses is difficult because of the vagaries of the intake. In 1865 Mr Bonham Carter, trying to do an analysis, said, 'There were great difficulties because probationers were selected to fill vacancies some of whom are considered to have completed their training though they have not.'[46] No doubt, pressed by the treasurer, Mrs Wardroper was taking on probationers as staff and filling vacancies as they occurred. It is for this reason that Mr Bonham Carter was always thwarted in his efforts to get an organised 'classing' system. Mrs Wardroper resisted to the end. It is also possible to come across names in reports and find that they are not on the main register.[47] These usually turn out to have been dismissed with more than usual alacrity.

Using the official register as a guide and excluding names that were only observers, there are 188 names in Book A for the nine-year period covering the stay at Surrey Gardens, and of these at least 62 did not complete their training. Of these 62 three died, two of typhoid and one of scarlet fever, seven 'resigned', usually no reason being given. Of the remaining 52 half were dismissed for misconduct – including three for insobriety, while the remainder were dismissed for 'poor health', often with the cryptic remark 'not strong enough for our work'. Sometimes the two categories overlap. For example, was 'want of energy' (a favourite of Mrs Wardroper's remarks) due to poor health or indolence? This means that a third did not survive their training year but this is conservative because some were dismissed before they reached the register.

The fact that so many were dismissed for glaring defects, including phthisis, indicates that either the selection was poor, the reference dishonest, or there was no choice. Unfortunately we do not know how many applications there were in the early years, but later Mrs Wardroper always boasted 'many applications'.

Professor Abel-Smith's comments that 'candidates for this arduous year were carefully selected by Mrs Wardroper' and 'a minimum educational attainment and maximum moral stature were essential requirements'[48] are not borne out by fact.

It is the sickness rate that is perhaps the most interesting. Candidates were supposed to have a signed medical certificate but some with tuberculosis and even syphilis seem to have slipped through the net.[49] If the recorded sickness is analysed – and probationers' letters home indicate that they often treated one another[50] – it will be seen to be closely related to working conditions. In this period there were 14 cases of diagnosed typhoid, typhus, scarlet fever and diphtheria, but another 15 were off with 'fever' and more than half were sick at some time with sore throats, diarrhoea and poisoned fingers. Perhaps most sadly ironic is the case of Elizabeth Pratt who during her training contracted both scarlet fever and diphtheria, and was then dismissed for 'poor health'. Harriet Turner, aged 23 years, died of scarlet fever and was buried in the Norwood cemetery at the expense of the Fund ('the sum not to exceed £5'). Not until Miss Nightingale started attacking 'the unhealthy plans' for the new St Thomas's was there any apparent contrition about sickness among the probationers.[51]

How this morbidity rate compares with females in similar age-specific groups and social class in the same period is difficult to tell, bearing in mind that the probationers were supposed to start with a clean bill of health. The rates are an improvement on those collected by Dr Farr for 1858 and published by Miss Nightingale in *Notes on Hospitals* (see Tables 3.1 and 3.2). The tables show a high rate due to zymotic disease in nurses compared with the female population of London. Taking the age group 20–45 years, according to Dr Farr's figures there were 34 deaths out of 262 nurses employed, which may explain why nine deaths at St Thomas's called for little comment.

Interestingly enough in the same period Sir James Paget analysed what had happened to 1,000 medical students who had been his pupils; 41 had died while still pupils, including 17 who died of phthisis, four at least caught fever while in hospital and two had committed suicide. Paget goes on to comment that the mortality rate 'agrees so nearly with the general average that it gives no reason for considering the medical profession to be either less or more than other pursuits, at least in its early stages'.[52]

The training period for medical students was four to five years and the 4.1 per cent mortality must be considered over this period. Taking a smaller sample of 300, 12 probationers seem to have died within four years of starting their training, so it appears as if the probationers had a similar mortality rate, and these rates were not particularly high compared with the age-specific mortality rate at the time. What Sir James omitted to mention was that they were probably high for the social group from which medical students were drawn.

However, it is not only the wastage during the training year that raises the question of Mrs Wardroper's judgement; if there was little choice and the applicants unsuitable a high drop out rate was inevitable. What was more disturbing was the fact that of the 126 'survivors' from the Surrey Gardens period no less than 12 were dismissed from their first post: two for insobriety, one sent as matron and one as a sister. Most of these 12 had good reports from Mrs Wardroper. A further 24 resigned and 'left the service' including a number who left because of ill health, two died and two went as patients into mental asylums. It is difficult to be sure how many ever received their third gratuity because the recording is haphazard, but a generous estimate is that out of a total of 188 only 50 were still in hospitals at the end of three years. After ten years of the scheme there were probably not more than 50 nurses with the Nightingale certificate in active work in hospitals for the poor sick.

What people think is happening is as important as what actually happened. The Fund Council was influential and articulate and its publicity was good. Men like Bonham Carter, Harry Verney and William Rathbone began to speak and write with authority on nursing matters. Within three years the Fund was being pressed to provide nurses for other hospitals. The most important request came from William Rathbone of Liverpool who had a profound respect for Miss Nightingale and later became a Council member, but Mr Rathbone with his long association with charity organisations thought that if he gave enough money a reformed nursing system could be introduced quickly. Miss Nightingale complained that Mr Rathbone 'pressed too hard', with the result that the two schemes for Liverpool[53] drained the

Table 3.1: Numbers and Ages of Matrons, Sisters, and Nurses (Living and Dying) in Fifteen London Hospitals (Names of the hospitals, – St Mary's; St George's; Westminster; Charing Cross; Middlesex; University College; Royal Free; Kings' College; St Bartholomew's; London; Guy's; St Thomas'; Small Pox; Fever; and Consumption)

LIVING (1858)

	Total			Specified Ages of Living, March, 1858											
	Total of all Ages	Ages Specified	Ages *not* Specified	Under 20	20	25	30	35	40	45	50	55	60	65	70 and up
Matrons, Sisters and Nurses	521	391	130	1	10	45	55	93	64	59	34	18	8	4	...
Matrons and Sisters	118	90	28	...	...	4	11	22	16	20	8	5	3	1	...
Nurses	403	301	102	1	10	4	44	71	48	39	26	13	5	3	...

Table 3.1: (continued)

DYING (1848–57)

| | Total | | | Ages of the Dying | | | | | | | | | | | |
	Total of all Ages	Ages Speci-fied	Ages *not* Spec-fied	Under 20	20	25	30	35	40	45	50	55	60	65	70 and up
Matrons, Sisters and Nurses	79	79	...	...	...	4	11	8	18	8	10	7	6	2	5
*Matrons and Sisters (so dis-tinguished	19	19	...	...	...	...	2	1	4	...	3	2	1	1	5
Nurses	60	60	...	...	...	4	9	7	14	8	7	5	5	1	...

*In the return of deaths, four Hospitals do not distinguish the Matrons and Sisters from the Nurses, and in this Table they are included with the Nurses.

Table 3.2: Table of the Mortality of Matrons, Sisters, and Nurses, at Different Ages, in Fifteen London Hospitals, compared with the Mortality of the Female Population of London

Ages	Matrons, Sisters and Nurses (1848–1857)		Female Population of London	
	Annual Rate of Mortality to 1000 living at the respective Ages			
	By *all* returned Diseases	By *Zymotic* Diseases	By *Zymotic* Diseases (1848–57)	By *all* returned Diseases (1848–54)
25 to 35	15.89	9.53	2.19	9.92
35–45	15.80	10.94	2.73	14.65
45–55	17.80	11.87	3.17	20.36
55–65	46.36	14.26	4.94	36.02

Fund of nurses in the early years. Apart from Liverpool, the Fund, partly because it needed the money, made arrangements with specially nominated candidates sent by institutions, such as Miss Rappe from Uppsala, Mrs Deeble from Netley and Jane Markham from Swansea. In these cases the Fund had little control over their appointments. Later Miss Nightingale regretted some of these arrangements because she considered hasty or shortened trainings were a poor advertisement for the Fund.

One of the hasty trainings Miss Nightingale regretted was that of Miss Osburn, who in 1867 was sent by special arrangement to Australia with a team of nurses that the Fund could ill afford to spare, because that year they sent Miss Torrance, one of the first Specials, and five nurses to the new St Pancras Infirmary at Highgate.[54] Once these commitments were honoured there were few Nightingale trained nurses for elsewhere. Contrary to popular belief only six who had done the training became superintendents before 1871 and only eight became sisters at St Thomas's; of these one was dismissed and at least three others were to earn Miss Nightingale's bitter execration.

In 1870 Mr Bonham Carter, who was not given to exaggeration, wrote to Mr Rathbone, 'we have hitherto turned out only two good superintendents', and with great perspicacity, 'we fail for want of good teachers.'[55] Correcting this failure was to be the main problem of the next decade.

Notes

1. Cook, Sir E., *The Life of Florence Nightingale,* vol. 2, p. 11.
2. Hon. Col. Grey to R. Baggallay, BL, Add Mss 45750, 22 December 1860, f. 3.
3. H. Bonham Carter to FN, GLRO, A/NFC/73/2, 6 June 1862.
4. *Nightingale Fund Council Report,* November 1862. (Signed Jebb, printed E. Faithful & Co.)
5. GLRO, HI/ST/NTS/AI/2; also HI/ST/NTS/C14.
6. GLRO, A/NFC/2/1, 1861–2.
7. FN to J. McNeill, GLRO, HI/ST/NC/2SU146, 22 April 1962.
8. Abel-Smith, B., *A History of the Nursing Profession* (Heinemann, London, 1960), p. 41.
9. *Statement of the Appropriation of the Fund* (Blades & Blades, March 1863), GLRO, HI/NTS/Y36, 2.
10. J. Sutherland to H. Bonham Carter, GLRO, HI/ST/NC/11 (n.d.).
11 H. Bonham Carter to Lord Beauchamp, GLRO, HI/ST/NC, 18/5, 20, 1 August 1872.
12. Cameron, H.C., *Mr Guy's Hospital* (Longmans, Green and Co., London, 1954), p. 195.
13. Bonham Carter, H., *Suggestions for Improving the Management of a Nursing Department of Large Hospitals* (pamphlet).
14. Lambert, R., *Sir John Simon 1816–1904* (MacGibbon & Kee, London, 1963), p. 478f.
15. FN to R. Baggallay, GLRO, HI/ST/NC1/63/1, 13 January 1863.
16. FN to H. Bonham Carter, GLRO, HI/ST/NC/18(6), 11 November 1865, 20 March 1865.
17. Sir H. Verney to H. Bonham Carter, GLRO, HI/ST/NC18(6), 11 November 1865.
18. FN to H. Bonham Carter, GLRO, HI/ST/NC18(6), 3 September 1865.
19. H. Bonham Carter to FN, GLRO, HI/ST/NC18(6), 17, 21 March 1865.
20. FN to H. Bonham Carter, GLRO, HI/ST/NC18(6), 14 September 1865.
21. R. Whitfield to H. Bonham Carter, GLRO, HI/ST/NC18(6), 10 April 1865.
22. Sir J. Clark to H. Bonham Carter, GLRO, HI/ST/NC18(6), 25 January 1866.
23. GLRO, A/NFC/16/5.
24. H. Bonham Carter to FN, BL, Add Mss 47714, 20 March 1865, f. 104.
25. R. Whitfield to H. Bonham Carter, GLRO, HI/ST/NC18(6), December 1865.
26. Sir J. Clark to H. Bonham Carter, GLRO, HI/ST/NC18(6), 40, 25 January 1866.
27. FN to H. Bonham Carter, BL, Add Mss 47714, 4 January 1866, f. 124-7.
28. *The Lancet,* 31 March 1866.
29. FN to H. Bonham Carter, BL, Add Mss 47715, 19 December 1867, f. 140 (also f. 41).
30. Nightingale Fund Council Minutes, 28 February 1867.

31. J. Carr to H. Bonham Carter, GLRO, HI/ST/NC18(7), 1 February 1860.
32. See Chapter 4.
33. To the Editor of *Macmillan's Magazine* from Florence Nightingale, BL, Add Mss 45800, April 1867, f. 91.
34. Regulations 1867, GLRO, HI/NTS/a2/3.
35. Mill, J.S., *Principles of Political Economy* (Longman, London, 1872).
36. *The Nightingale Fund Council Annual Abstract of Accounts*, 1872.
37. *Recollections of Rachel Strong*, GLRO, HI/ST/NTS/Y/15.
38. GLRO, HI/ST, A106/2, Unpublished thesis, quoted in Granshaw, L.
39. Strong, R. *Reminiscences* (privately printed), 1935.
40. GLRO, HI/ST/NC18(1)5, July 1863.
41. FN to R.G. Whitfield, BL, Add Mss, March 1863, f. 34.
42. Cope, Z., *Florence Nightingale and the Doctors* (Museum, London, 1954), p. 112.
43. Parsons, F., *History of St. Thomas's Hospital* (Methuen, London, 1936), vol. 3, pp. 155–9.
44. Ibid.
45. S.E. Wardroper to H. Bonham Carter, GLRO, HI/ST/NC18(4), 14 March 1864.
46. H. Bonham Carter to FN, GLRO, HI/ST/NC18(20)1 (n.d.).
47. The Red Register – not all the names entered in the working register are entered in the Red Book. GLRO, HI/ST/NTS/C1.
48. Abel-Smith, B., *A History of the Nursing Profession* (Heinemann, London, 1960), p. 21.
49. FN to H. Bonham Carter, BL, Add Mss 47718, 1873, f. 92.
50. The Cadbury Letters. Mary Cadbury's letters home giving a graphic description of the probationers treating one another's septic fingers and Mrs Cadbury sending her daughter ointment with which to treat friends.
51. FN to H. Bonham Carter, BL, Add Mss 47717 (1873), f. 198.
52. *St Bartholomew's Hospital Gazette*, 1869. Article by Sir James Paget quoted by Graham Grant University Health Services, Newcastle-on-Tyne – letter to *The Times*, 13 January 1983.
53. See Chapter 5.
54. Ibid.
55. H. Bonham Carter to Wm. Rathbone, GLRO, HI/ST/NC18(11), 1 October 1870.

4. Training Midwifery Nurses

But with all their defects, midwifery statistics point to one truth, namely that there is a large amount of preventable mortality in midwifery practice, and that, as a general rule, the mortality is far, far greater in lying-in hospitals than among lying-in at home... One feels disposed to ask whether it can be true that, in the hands of educated accoucheurs, the inevitable fate of women undergoing, not a diseased but an entirely natural condition, at home, is that one out of every 128 must die?

Florence Nightingale, Notes on Lying-In Institutions, *1871*

In pre-Christian times pregnant women prayed to Diana, Juno and Isis for safe delivery, for from time immemorial attendance at childbirth has been considered 'women's business'.[1] Traditionally women have always cultivated the healing arts and in medieval Europe women practised both medicine and surgery.[2] However, in the thirteenth century with the development of the barber surgeon guilds, the surgeons drew apart, and in the towns where the guilds operated surgeons had the exclusive rights to use instruments; although some women were admitted their numbers were few.[3] This development had important consequences for midwives for although (until the invention of forceps in the seventeenth century) surgeons could do little, the practice was to send for a surgeon when normal delivery was not possible.

In seventeenth-century England most normal midwifery was carried out by women, and some were educated and rose to fame and even to fortune, although many midwives remained ignorant, with practices allied with superstitions. As early as 1616 a group of midwives supported by Dr Peter Chamberlen, of the forceps family fame, mounted a campaign for a system of instruction and secular regulation and asked the King for a Charter.[4] Unfortunately the petition was opposed by the physicians, some of whom were beginning to find that the practice of midwifery could be lucrative.

The eighteenth century saw the decline of the midwife and the emergence of the man-midwife, a doctor undertaking, and often specialising in, normal midwifery for gain. This affected the status of midwives and the attraction of midwifery at a time when industrialisation and the increase in the population made their services more urgent. At the same time women were deprived of another traditional way of earning their living, for with increasing industrialisation which so often separated the workshop from the home, much gainful employ was lost to women tied to their home and family. Even if women were not so tied, many occupations that were once feminine prerogatives like women's hairdressing and stay making had passed to men.[5] It was in this social and occupational climate where fewer women, and certainly fewer educated women, worked outside the home that the campaigns for the reform of nursing and midwifery were launched in the nineteenth century.

In spite of the interventions of the better-paid man-midwife with his instruments, Dr Charles White pointed out that

> Although the poor were half starved and diseased and served only by ignorant midwives their maternal death rate might be less than that of patients delivered in lying-in hospitals, or of the more affluent class attended by men.[6]

The lying-in hospitals of the eighteenth century were plagued by puerperal sepsis and for this reason the new charity hospitals often refused to have maternity wards. An exception was the Middlesex Hospital in 1747 but even here the idea had to be abandoned. In 1752 the General Lying-in Hospital (later knows as Queen Charlotte's) was founded but in common with other such hospitals it was subject to a high death-rate from puerperal infection. Many people, including Miss Nightingale, doubted whether maternity hospitals ought to exist.[7] This raised problems as to where midwives, male and female, could, or should, be trained.

Miss Nightingale gave much thought to the subject and, true to her sanitary principles, she believed that the high death-rate could be prevented and turned her attention to using part of the Nightingale Fund for training persons from country parishes as midwifery nurses for the poor sick. In contrast to the prevailing view among most doctors, Miss Nightingale held that the midwife 'proper' should be capable of dealing with all cases, including those of difficulty, and that her training should not be less than two years as was in the case on the continent. In 1861 she wrote to her friend Harriet Martineau: 'In nearly every country but our own there is a Government School for Midwives. I trust our School may lead the way towards supplying a long felt want in England.'[8] The scheme Miss Nightingale had in mind had a two-fold purpose: to give the rural poor a service, and to pave the way for a national midwifery training under government control. Like the scheme at St Thomas's it was to be a prototype.

Her choice for a training school fell on King's College Hospital with which she had a close relationship. Her old friend Mr William Bowman was on the staff, and it was he who in 1848 had been largely instrumental in the foundation of the St John's House scheme for training nurses. The superintendence was now under Mary Jones – Miss Nightingale's 'dearest friend' – who was responsible for the nursing services at King's College Hospital. In the same letter to Harriet Martineau Miss Nightingale says that Miss Jones was 'certainly the best moral trainer of women I know'. However, although the governors were co-operative and Miss Nightingale was sure that the 'moral atmosphere would be such that any mother could trust her daughter there', the scheme had disadvantages: King's College Hospital was poor. In April 1862 Miss Nightingale writing to Sir J. McNeill, explained:

> K.C.H. is so poor that although it generously gives the services of its offi-cers gratuitously (except for the midwife who is ours) it is unable to pay anything towards the beds. We are unable to board our probationers quite as gratuitously as we do at St Thomas's.[9]

According to Mr Bonham Carter in his summary of the work of the Fund written in 1913, an agreement was reached with the governors in 1860.[10] But the first discussion by the committee of the Fund seems to have been in October 1861 when a letter from Miss Nightingale was read and it was agreed that the secretary should draw up a contract with St John's House and that £500 a year should be authorised to pay training expenses.[11] This would seem to indicate that either Mr Bonham Carter's memory was at fault, or that in spite of her illness in 1860 Miss Nightingale, when she wished, held the reins of the Fund in her own hands. In the agreement the Nightingale Fund, 'furnished and maintained 10 lying-in beds in a capacious ward set aside'. On the other hand the Fund did not pay fees, what *The Lancet* called 'douceurs', to hospital officers who helped with the training. At King's College such services were free. The Fund paid £12 for each pupil in advance to the hospital to offset the cost of board and lodging for the six-months' course, and the pupils received no salary during that time. The annual reports for the period 1862-67 are not explicit about the number of pupils trained but other sources suggested that the vacan-cies were never filled. Nor do the accounts show how the money was spent; Professor Smith extrapolating from the payments in 1864 thinks that the total number of pupils trained in the five years was about 30.[12] If this is so, allowing generously for the salary and board of Miss Yate, the midwifery teacher, it looks as if the Fund were paying over £300 a year – almost a quarter of its available income – to King's College to maintain ten beds.

The regulations for the pupils were different from those for the probationers at St Thomas's Hospital. In the first place the pupils had to accept the rules of the St John's sisterhood: 'The pupils while under training will readily and cheerfully obey the rules of St. John's House.' Once her six-months' training was completed the pupil had to sign that she would 'continue to employ herself for four years under the direction of the Managers (the employers who had sent her) attending such cases of confinements and sickness as the Managers shall select among the poor of..... and the immediate neighbourhood'.[13] The blank space was filled in with the name of the parish, district or estate sending the midwife. It was, in fact, a contract *à trois* (The Fund, the nurse, and the employer) in which the employer had to promise to continue to employ the midwife at a salary of at least £20 a year, and to provide comfortable lodgings for four years, provided of course that the midwife gave satisfactory service. Learning by their difficulties at St Thomas's the Fund inserted a penalty clause into the contract:

> If she [the midwife] give up her engagement to marry or voluntarily do anything which shall prevent or interfere with the proper discharge of her duties, she shall repay to the Managers, by way of penalty, the sum of £40 less £5 for every complete year during which she shall have been employed, such sum to be recoverable as liquidated damages.

There is no information as to whether this clause was ever enforced.

The other innovation at King's College Hospital was that there were definite entry dates for pupils twice a year with what Mr Bonham Carter called 'classing'. The Fund achieved with Miss Jones what they failed to do with Mrs Wardroper. Unfortunately the records do not show how many people completed their contract and where they went. In 1863 the Fund's annual report stated that

> the plan for midwifery training at King's College Hospital for nurses to be employed among the poor was making progress... the probationers who had been sent out from hence as trained Nurses were employed in country parishes and giving satisfaction.[14]

Hereafter, references to the scheme are more guarded but the 1866 report provides a clue to one source of supply and that was the Parochial Mission Women Association. Apparently the managers of the Association provided the cost of the nurses' maintenance while under training and guaranteed their subsequent employment. The same report stresses the urgent need for proper nursing for women during their confinements and for their infants:

> The poor are now almost entirely without skilled nursing in this respect, and the want is not met by the attendance of medical men. In those places where nurses have been established they are admitted by the parish doctors to be not only a boon to the poor, but a great assistance to medical men themselves.[15]

The last statement is not merely publicity but is borne out by many of the letters requesting the training of midwives. The overwhelming impression is of poverty, particularly rural poverty, and harassed clergymen without funds doing their best for a poor parish. If the need was so great, the question has to be asked, why wasn't the response to the scheme better?

One suspects, and the Fund probably realised, that those in the greatest need could not get help. However meagre their earnings at this time, midwives could not forgo them for six months, and poor parishes could not subsidise their midwives; nor could they with the ups and downs of the depression, guarantee to pay the midwife on her return. Miss Nightingale, with great prescience unusual at that time, realised that the problem was beyond charity and that government intervention was necessary.[16]

In spite of the execration she was to suffer later Miss Jones seems to have been remarkably tolerant and flexible in dealing with the individual needs of midwives and their families. Those like Mrs Tilt, for example, who had a young baby of her own, were allowed to bring the baby and arrangements were made for its care. In the early days Miss Jones earned the approbation of the Fund Council and Sir John Clark wrote that his father, Sir James, approved of the arrangements and 'he thinks that Miss Jones will catch better fish than poor Mrs Wardroper with mere words'.[17] However, all was not well, for in spite of acting on Chadwick's advice and appealing to the Boards of Guardians to send candidates for training and advertisements in *The Times* addressed especially to the clergy, the scheme did not attract enough candidates. The Fund might have weathered this for a year or so but it soon became clear that there were other problems relating to the arrangements at King's College Hospital.

In her *Notes on Different Systems of Nursing*[18] Miss Nightingale commended the system where 'nurses belong to a religious organisation and are under their own spiritual head, the institution being administered by a separate, secular governing body'. In this system, she maintained, there was a higher than average care of the sick and a higher universal sense of morality. Her *bête noire* was the system in which the head of the religious order also administered the institution. In her devotion to her 'dear old friend' Mr Bowman, and her enthusiasm for 'dearest friend' Mary Jones, she put King's College Hospital into category one, though, be it noted, she had turned down attempts by Herbert and Bowman to start the main nurse training school there.

St John's House had been founded in 1848, so named because it originated in the parish of St John in Fitzroy Square, and was nominally under the aegis of the Bishop of London. Like the nurses under Miss Sellon and the Bishop of Exeter it had a strong Tractarian background. The institute was run by a Master who was a clergyman and a Lady Superintendent whose aim was to raise the character and improve the qualifications of nurses by providing moral and religious instruction. Membership of St John's was divided into three classes:

1. Probationers who had a two-year training in hospitals before becoming nurses.
2. Nurses who nursed in hospitals and in patients' homes and who were paid wages.
3. Sisters who instructed the probationers and who did some nursing.[19]

No group took vows. St John's and similar institutions provided trained nurses to hospitals for a fixed sum and several hospitals, such as the Westminster, saw this arrangement as an advantage. Miss Jones became superintendent in 1854, and was thus responsible for supplying a team of six for Scutari. Then in 1856 she brought a team of nurses to King's College Hospital and took over the responsibility for the nursing service.

Mary Jones was a remarkable woman and was perhaps the greatest inspiration to Miss Nightingale, who consulted her on all nursing matters. Although Florence Nightingale herself is regarded as the main advisor to William Rathbone's plans for nursing in Liverpool, probably the most practical advisor was Mary Jones. At King's College Hospital she and her sisters were responsible for the domestic management and the catering; they improved the conditions for patients, their diets, the hygiene and they succeeded in preventing drunkenness among patients. At the same time they started a planned training system for probationers. The superintendent and the sisters constituted an autonomous service within the hospital; they worked with the doctors but were not *under* the doctors. In the 1860s, apart from their work at King's College and Charing Cross, the sisters were serving 4,000 meals to the poor Out Patients from King's College daily and visiting their homes regularly. It was a remarkable comprehensive and integrated nursing service. The sisters also worked in the London docks during the cholera epidemic and in Staffordshire with typhoid cases, with at least two dying in the course of their duty.[20] Mary Jones was well placed to advise on Liverpool.

The disadvantage of the sisterhoods was that the Oxford Movement, as the Tractarians became called, aroused deep-seated fears in certain staunch Protestants; Lord Shaftesbury was almost fanatical in his denunciation and, with several conversions to Rome like Newman and Manning, suspicions increased. The arrangements at King's College Hospital were delicate for peace had to be kept between the requirements of St John's House – especially the Master, the largely Protestant Board of Governors and the Nightingale Fund Council.

Although there were some difficulties during the first year or two, peace apparently reigned and there was little correspondence; then in 1866 dissension broke out between the Master, the Reverend Giraud, and Miss Jones. During this period Miss Jones and Miss Nightingale were in constant communication on both professional and personal matters and Miss Jones was a frequent visitor to Miss Nightingale. It was this conflict with the chaplain that caused Miss Nightingale to write the much quoted letter:

> The whole reform of nursing both at home and abroad has consisted of this. To take all power out of the hands of men and put into one female trained head and make her responsible for everything – regarding the internal management and discipline being carried out... Don't let the Doctor make himself the Head Nurse, and there is no worse matron than the Chaplain.[21]

However, not content with fighting for control over the nurses without interference from the chaplain Miss Jones conceived a new plan, to make herself the spiritual as well as the nursing head. This was not so outrageous as Professor Smith suggests since some sisterhoods were being formed with a Mother Superior. However, the suggestion that an altar be set up and the sacrament exposed was unwise and brought a protest from the governors and Bishop Tait of London. This was taking Anglicanism too far. At this stage Miss Jones offered to sever her connection with St. John's and to take her sisters with her.[22] This filled Miss Nightingale with alarm. 'I should think it would be the greatest calamity that has happened in all my unfortunate life if you and the sisters seceded leaving the nurses and K.C.H. in the hands of St. John's.' Then she threatened, 'if Miss Jones goes I will take our midwifery school away and bestow it wherever she goes'.[23] The attraction of King's College Hospital for the midwifery scheme was apparently not the St John's system but Miss Jones as the superintendent.

In November 1867 Miss Jones offered her resignation without apparently consulting Miss Nightingale. This brought an eight-page letter in pencil to Mr Bowman in which Miss Nightingale exhorts him to 'Burn' but in another place 'return to me'. Fortunately for the records Mr Bowman 'returned'. From this letter the course of events that led to the final showdown can be construed. It would appear that at some stage the Bishop of London had at least given the 'Mother Superior' idea some consideration and the Fund Council had tried to get a reconciliation by suggesting amended rules. However, Miss Nightingale had been obliged to tell Miss Jones that when they came the revised rules did not embody all the Fund's suggestions. At the same time Miss Nightingale had received complaints from the governors that Miss Jones was a secret Roman Catholic, which Miss Jones had countered with a statement to show that she had been traduced, and she suspected that this included mistrust by Mr Bowman. Miss Nightingale continued that she was not supporting Miss Jones, whom she obviously thought was acting foolishly, but to plead for leniency and to show her state of mind and to ask for allowances. At this point Mr Bowman added his own comment in pencil on the returned letter which was, 'I do make allowances if only she would hold on and let the points be discussed a while', which seems to suggest that Miss Jones was indeed in an excitable and unreasonable state of mind. Miss Nightingale ends the letter significantly: 'I look upon this crisis as one of deeper importance than you or even Miss Jones do. I look upon it *that sisterhoods are from henceforth impossible.* God help you.'[24] Help that no doubt Mr Bowman felt he needed.

When Miss Jones and her sisters left the governors considered asking the Clewer sisters of Berkshire but they were associated with Miss Twining whose ideas on nursing were incompatible with those of Miss Nightingale. The Bishop then suggested the Deaconesses led by the Reverend Pelham Dale, but this was even less acceptable and in the end the governors made a deal with the All Saints sisterhood, who were already supplying University College Hospital, without consulting the Nightingale Fund. This was the last straw, and the Fund withdrew the training school.[25] Miss Nightingale was bitter:

> The training at K.C.H. is now as bad or worse (as I am informed) and the Bishop is consecrating the nursing which leads to the Church yards with as much apparent zeal as Bishops are said to consecrate the Church itself. There is no other remedy possible except for the hospital to break their contract with St. John's Council... I am waiting to reopen the midwifery school till I can reconstitute it elsewhere under Miss Jones.[26]

Throughout the spring of 1868 there was a brisk correspondence between Mr Bowman and Miss Nightingale, with Mr Bowman explaining that the attraction of St John's was that it saved money because the Lady Probationers paid for their board. In fact finance lay at the root of many of the problems. In March of 1866 *The Lancet* had criticised the Fund for spending £350 maintaining patients and hoped that 'the Committee would spread its benefits over several hospitals'.[27] Somewhat belatedly Miss Nightingale now suggested that the Fund could be in trouble with its subscribers. But at its back the Fund must have heard the demands of the new St Thomas's Hospital and the 'hard bargain'.

As passions cooled it was decided to put a good face on it and for the governors to put out a statement that

> the primary object had been carried out successfully, but that the governors had felt anxiety about outbreaks of puerperal fever, and on the advice of Dr Priestly, had decided to close the ward at the end of 1867.[28]

This did not satisfy Miss Nightingale because, as she said, it looked as if the governors were the only ones who took alarm about the deaths and she had 'never ceased to try and obtain information and also to draw up comparative statistics with lying-in wards in London, Paris and Dublin'.[29] However, having said that there had been 28 deaths out of 792 deliveries, neither the Fund nor the governors were on strong ground for imputing the reason for closure to the puerperal death-rate; 35 per 1,000 was not exceptional for a lying-in hospital or ward; for example, during this period there was a rise to 44 per 1,000 at Guy's and there was no question of closing the ward.[30] Undoubtedly the reason for the withdrawal of the School was the dispute over the position of Miss Jones, which Miss Nightingale saw as a matter of principle – the matron must be supreme in nursing matters. Second, and to a lesser extent, there was the question of money. Spending nearly a quarter of their income maintaining ten maternity beds was perhaps not the best way of the Fund using its money.

The dispute is important and there are conclusions to be drawn from it, though not necessarily those drawn by Professor Smith, that Miss Nightingale lied in order to exercise power and that she was jealous of any attempt at improvements other than her own.[31] Rather the opposite, all her life she had been strongly, and often excessively, attracted to certain individuals and, as Jowett was to point out, she was prone to exaggerate. Hyperbole gave weight to her utterances and made them more colourful, though not necessarily more accurate. Having invested approval and admiration she often remained stubbornly loyal in spite of evidence that suggested that there might be an element of clay in the feet of the idol. This was to happen in the cases of Mrs Wardroper, Mr Whitfield, Miss Torrance, Miss Williams and many others. In spite of her ability to see to the heart of the matter and to analyse it in an objective manner, when it came to dealing with people her heart often ruled her head. It did so in the case of Mary Jones, because her past experience in the Crimea had warned her against basing her scheme for nurse training on a religious order, and yet in the case of St John's House she was saying that in 1861 they were providing the best nursing in London and she was willing to take the risk. When she could no longer close her eyes to the basic defect which she had so acutely analysed in 1855, she wrote 'sisterhoods are henceforth impossible'. She had learned her lesson and she never tried again. The episode is important because when the great schism came with St Thomas's in the 1870s, taking the training away and joining it to a sisterhood was an option now closed to her.

The concern for maternal deaths from infection and the lack of skilled midwifery for the poor was not perfunctory. Together with Dr Sutherland she started to collect statistics and in 1871 she published *The Introductory Notes on Lying-in Hospitals Together with a Proposal for Organising an Institution for Training Midwives and Midwifery Nurses.*[32] In this pamphlet Miss Nightingale argues that the high mortality rate could be prevented by better sanitation, ventilation and less crowding. Her reason for suggesting this was, of course, that it would prevent the transference of miasma. In arguing the right thing for wrong reason the book undoubtedly made a contribution to the thinking on the subject at that time.

In 1867 when the school at King's College Hospital closed the Nightingale Fund reported that 'Although the School for Midwifery Nurses is at present in abeyance, the Committee hope to be able to re-establish it elsewhere.' It was always among the long-term aims of the Fund to do for midwives what it was doing for nurses, but for a variety of reasons this never proved possible.

When Mary Jones wrote to Bishop Tait that her only course was to sever her connection with St John's House, she and six sisters left to form their own sisterhood. Florence Nightingale was against such a hazardous enterprise; nevertheless she gave it her support and a donation trusting in Mary Jones as 'having the firmest and clearest mind I know'.

The new sisterhood was founded with its constitution in 1868 as the Community of St Mary and St John the Evangelist with a rule based on that of St Augustine. Florence Nightingale urged them to undertake Poor Law Infirmary nursing; however Mary Jones said she was too old, but that she would start a hospital on her own. After many difficulties and moves she succeeded in establishing a small hospital in Kensington Square, St Joseph's Hospital for Incurables, which took in patients for whom there was no known cure. Duly blest by the Bishop of London, Mary died in 1887 from typhoid, the 'friend of God'. The foundation was destined eventually to become St Mary's Convent and Nursing Home in Chiswick still doing sterling work and having celebrated its centenary in 1996.[33]

After 1867 Miss Nightingale continued to consider the future for midwifery, but in arguing that midwifery should be a career for educated women able to undertake all cases she immediately ran into the vexed question of the admission of women to the profession of medicine. If educated women were to be trained to a high standard to be midwives what was the difference between them and the man-midwife doctor? In 1865, while the scheme at King's College was in progress, the Ladies Medical College was set up; its long-term aim was the admission of women to medicine, but its immediate objective was the rehabilitation of midwifery as an occupation for gentlewomen.[34] The prospectus and curriculum were sent to the Fund and its backing sought and Lord Houghton, a Fund trustee and committee member, was on the College Council. Although the aim of the Society for Midwifery appeared to be identical with Miss Nightingale's own, she was nevertheless far from encouraging and was rather sarcastic about Lord Houghton's participation. One reason seemed to be that she still had ideas about founding a Midwifery College on the continental pattern and training Physician-Acchoucheuses - though she had been warned by Dr Blackwell that even in France and Germany midwives were being restricted to routine practice and the better-off cases were passing to men.[35] Probably the real reason for her lack of enthusiasm about the College was the fact that she was almost obsessional about women wasting themselves wanting to do medicine when there was so much to do without fighting men: 'would we could induce the women doctors to take up midwifery and nursing while they are moving heaven and earth to go in for ordinary men's examinations'.[36]

In spite of her clarity of vision on many matters Miss Nightingale was often contradictory and confused about women's emancipation. Her formative years were before the agitation for women's rights, and she had, as she said, worked and exercised power without a vote. Her social position and the fact she had a private income of over £500 a year must have affected her attitude to the aspiration of middle-class women without these two assets. They needed the money.

As well as producing a training that would give a safe midwifery service there was the question of how many grades were needed. In

England there were midwives, monthly nurses, and what the Fund called 'Midwifery nurses'. Miss Nightingale therefore enquired what was happening in other countries to whom she sent elaborate questionnaires. The reply from Dr Gottwald of the Midwives Clinique, Berlin, who dutifully filled in the 28 sections, showed that in Germany they only trained one grade of midwife who, after a five-month course for which she paid a substantial fee, took a qualifying examination and then practised according to the *Lehrbuch*.[37] The course appears to have been more academic than that offered by the Fund, but less rigorous than the course at the Medical Ladies College. It was this standard pattern of midwifery training in the Austro-German Empire that appealed to Miss Nightingale, and with which, in the end, the Central Midwives Board had some affinity.

An early attempt to obtain the regulation of midwifery had been made in 1826 by the formation of the Obstetrical Society, and in 1872 in order to meet the growing demand for training and control of midwifery the Society proposed holding its own examinations, its proposals being sent to the Nightingale Fund.[38] The Society planned to hold examinations four times a year and candidates wishing to take these had to submit a certificate of moral character and evidence that they had attended 25 labours under supervision. The examinations were to cover the anatomy of the female pelvis, mechanisms, the course and management of natural labour, indications of abnormalities, the emergencies that may occur, a general knowledge of the puerperal state, and the duties of the midwife in seeking medical aid. The successful midwife would receive a Diploma certifying that she was a skilled midwife, competent to attend natural labour.

This also met with Miss Nightingale's withering disapproval. In a letter to Dr Sutherland she wrote: 'This is a first attempt, but what an attempt, as if any educated midwife would come forward for such a certificate.'[39] Professor Smith sees Miss Nightingale's failure to give this scheme support as part of 'her own failure with midwives training which impelled her to thwart the plans of others',[40] but her rejection is in keeping with her attitude to nurse training in general. First, she was against certificates and registration, which was the aim of the Society, because they were meaningless, though she did admit that the case for registration in midwifery could be different because it was a circumscribed field. Second, she knew all too well of how little value were certificates of 'moral character' or 'having attended 25 deliveries'. Third, and most important, the Society did not offer a training and it was the *sine qua non* of the Nightingale doctrine that trained nurses and midwives must have undergone formal instruction. Finally, and most objectional, there was the proposal to make the General Medical

Council responsible for the registration of midwives with the power to grant licences, on a yearly basis, and the power to strike off names. This would have placed midwives under the control of another profession and under the jurisdiction of a group that were in fact their rivals for midwifery practice and who had a vested interest in keeping midwives in a lowly place and in restricting their earning capacity.[41]

Dr Henry Acland, Regius Professor of Medicine at Oxford, member of the General Medical Council, and a friend of the Nightingale family, got in touch with Miss Nightingale on the subject. In 1869 the General Medical Council made tentative proposals for granting certificates to the various occupations connected with medicine, including midwifery. The medical profession were divided as the whether they should try to control midwifery as a 'necessary evil' until it withered away (replaced, as in America, by qualified medical practitioners), or whether such a task was beneath its dignity. Miss Nightingale replied to Dr Acland courteously but firmly that

> experience teaches me that nursing and medicine must never be mixed up. It spoils both... if I were not afraid of being misunderstood I would say that the less knowledge of medicine that the hospital matron has the better (1) because it does not improve her sanitary practice, (2) because it would make her miserable and intolerable to the doctors.[42]

This is an interesting insight into Miss Nightingale's idea of the role of nurses and why she was not keen on doctor's lectures even for the Specials. Nursing was more than being an assistant to the doctor and it included being a 'sanitary missioner' and a health educator, an art, she implies, the nurse would not learn from the doctor.

In spite of this refusal, Dr Acland, who became chairman of the General Medical Council, continued to explore the possibility of the Council becoming the registering body for what were later called paramedical professions. In 1873 Dr Acland sent out draft proposals for Miss Nightingale's consideration; these were presumably from the committee that had been set up to enquire into its powers to register women as midwives, nurses and dispensers.[43] Miss Nightingale's copy has added her red pencil marginalia which indicated her disapproval though she did suggest that midwives and dispensers could be in a different category from nurses. Time and again she and Mr Bonham Carter were to hammer home the difference between 'registering' a person to perform a specific function and from trying to measure, and register, an art. While she was not against the registration of midwives in 1873, Miss Nightingale thought it inappropriate for nurses and, thanks to the General Medical Council, the two issues were now mixed. Miss Nightingale questioned whether Dr Acland had enough evidence to give advice to the Council and Mr Bonham Carter agreed and wrote:

> I venture to think that in the present condition of knowledge (or igno-
> rance) which exists with regard to a proper system of training, and the
> very defective means of training at all, the time is not ripe for action on
> the part of the Council.[44]

From this it is clear that neither Miss Nightingale nor Mr Bonham Carter, nor presumably the Fund Council, were satisfied with the arrangements for nurse training by 1873 and that they regarded them as experimental and not as a blueprint for the future.

The enquiry on the part of the General Medical Council was in vain because it was shown that the Council did not have the power to register other bodies. The members were now not concerned with nurses, for like Miss Nightingale they considered that improvement could progress without registration, but there remained the problem of the midwife. The nub of the question was what was to be the status of the midwife; would she in fact take over most normal midwifery, or would the medical profession ultimately become responsible for the whole of the midwifery service? Until these questions were decided it was not possible to devise a training system and find an institution – not necessarily a hospital – to give it. To talk about 'registering' midwives before there were means to train them was putting the cart before the horse.

Dr Acland and Miss Nightingale continued to correspond and the Fund was still interested in midwifery training. Dr Acland had given qualified support to women doctors because the question was closely bound up with the need for educated women to attend child birth, but by 1876 it looks as if he had come round to Miss Nightingale's view on the subject because in reply to a letter from him she says, 'But we can't *make* them take up midwifery by legislating to prevent them from being doctors, let them train and let the market decide.'[45] Later in the same letter she says 'but no woman shall practise midwifery unless she has passed an examination, but where is the training School for Midwives?' By this time the Medical Ladies College had been superseded by the School of Medicine for Women which aimed at training women for the practice of medicine. It looks as if Miss Nightingale was bowing to events and the inevitability of women doctors. Her solution to the midwifery problem was that the government should act and until they did 'a vast field of women's work is left untilled, and a vast amount of suffering amongst the poor (and the rich too) is left unremedied.'[46]

In the same year Mr Bonham Carter was writing to George Frere of the St John's Maternity Scheme and looking at the proposed plan put up for a training school by the St John's Council: 'Nearer the time when the plans are ready the Nightingale Fund Council will be glad to avail themselves of its resource for the training of midwifery nurses for the poor.'[47] Nothing seems to have come of this, but later, in 1882, the Fund Council did give consideration to training midwives at St Marylebone where they had a training school for nurses.[48] However, it seems likely at this stage, unless they agreed to spend capital, that the Fund did not have the resources for further ventures.

In 1881 the initiative for the registration of midwives came from another source; the Matron's Aid Society became the Midwives Institute and then operated as a pressure group for the training and registration of midwives. Parliamentary Bills were drafted but they were all lost at various stages, mainly due to opposition from sections of the medical profession. As the Midwives Institute pressed for legislation so their cause was taken up by that active proponent of registration for nurses, Mrs Bedford Fenwick, but the institute, in spite of its small numbers, remained doggedly independent, believing, and rightly so, that there was more support for the registration of midwives than there was for nurses. Eventually the first Midwives Act was passed in 1902 'to secure the better training of midwives and to regulate their practice'. By now Miss Nightingale was no longer active, but it is significant that in 1903 the Fund Council considered an extension of the Nightingale School to include midwives although it was agreed that this did not come within the objects of the Trust and there was no way of altering the objects except with the assistance of the Charity Commission. It would however be possible to apply the Fund to the 'protection and sustenance of nurses who propose to qualify as midwives'.[49] This is in fact what the Fund did in the twentieth century; it funded certain Nightingale nurses to take the training of the Central Midwives Board.

The Nightingale Fund's experiment with 'midwifery nurse' training was on the whole disappointing. It is doubtful whether it produced more than 40 nurses for the poor sick. This was not necessarily the fault of the training but the fact that there was not enough money available, too few candidates could afford the training and there were too few parishes who could sponsor. Miss Nightingale was right when she divined that what was needed was government intervention. Moreover, the experiment did not pave the way to a Midwives College and training and education for what Miss Nightingale called 'real midwives' and above all for their registration and control. However, the scheme did receive publicity and it helped to focus the public's and the medical profession's mind on the urgent need for the training of midwives. The fact that it was another 40 years before there was a

Midwives Act in England is perhaps some indication that the experiment was ahead of its time.

Notes

1. Donnison, J., *Midwives and Medical Men* (Heinemann Educational Books, London 1977), p. 1.
2. Baly, M.E., *Nursing and Social Change* (Heinemann Medical Books, London, 1980), pp. 21–6.
3. Donnison, *Midwives*, p. 2.
4. Ibid., p. 13.
5. Ibid., p. 37.
6. McMath, J., *The Expert Midwife and a Treatise of the Diseases of Women with Child and in Childbed*, quoted in Donnison, p. 35.
7. Abel-Smith, B., *The Hospitals* (Heinemann, London, 1960), p. 23.
8. FN to H. Martineau, BL, Add Mss 45788, 24 September 1861, f. 131.
9. FN to Sir J. McNeill, BL, Add Mss 45768, 22 April, f. 172.
10. A summary of the work of the Nightingale Fund Council written by Henry Bonham Carter in 1913, GLRO, A/NFC/23.
11. Minutes of the NFC, October 1861, GLOR, A/NFC.2.1.
12. Smith, B.F., *Florence Nightingale – Reputation and Power* (Croom Helm, London, 1982), p. 160.
13. Regulations for Midwives, GLRO, HI/ST/NC18/1; see also BL, Add Mss 47714, August 1863, f. 15.
14. *Nightingale Fund Council Report*, 1863, para 3.
15. Ibid., 1866.
16. Donnison, *Midwives*, p. 88f.
17. Sir J. Clark to H. Bonham Carter, GLRO, HI/ST/NC18/3, n.d. (1863?).
18. Nightingale F., *Notes on Hospitals*, Appendix, pp. 181-7. (Longmans, Green & Co., London, 1863). See also separate pamphlet, *Notes on Different Systems of Nursing* (printed by Harrison & Sons).
19. Preface to the Annals of St. John's House, GLRO.
20. Myers, P. *Building for the Future – A Nursing History 1896 to 1996 to Commemorate the Centenary of St Mary's Convent Nursing Home Chiswick* St Mary's Convent, Chiswick, London University Printing Services,1996.
21. FN to M. Jones, GLRO, HI/ST/NC1/67(25), 1 May 1867. See also Abel-Smith, *A History*, p. 25.
22. FN's pencil memo on the dispute at KCH and the intervention of the Bishop? to J. Sutherland. BL, Add Mss 45752, 7 September 1867, f. 237.
23. FN to H. Verney, BL, Add Mss 45752, 13 October 1867, f. 240.
24. FN to Wm. Bowman, BL, Add Mss 45800, 22 December 1867, f. 193.
25. FN to J. Sutherland, BL, Add Mss 45752, 12 November 1867, f. 239 and f. 253.
26. FN to Wm. Bowman, BL, Add Mss 45800, 12 January 1868, f. 207.
27. *The Lancet*, 31 March 1866.

28. Statement from W. Powell Committee of Management KCH, BL. Add Mss 45800, February 1868, f. 217.
29. FN to J. Sutherland, BL, Add Mss 45800, 12 March 1868, f. 213.
30. *Guy's Hospital Gazette* (ed. Hander, C.E.) (BOSP, London), p. 193.
31. Smith, B.F., *Florence Nightingale*, pp. 162–3.
32. Nightingale F., *Notes on Lying-in Institutions* (Longmans, Green & Co., London, 1871) (HI/ST/NC4/66/20).
33. Ibid., Chapter 3.
34. Donnison, *Midwives*, p. 73.
35. Ibid., quoting from Eliz. Blackwell to FN, p. 85.
36. FN to J. Sutherland, GLRO, HI/ST/NC1/72, 16 April 1872.
37. FN to Dr Gottwald Frau Littra, GLRO, HI/ST/NC1/SU/72/4, 26 April 1872.
38. *Prospectus of the Obstetrical Society*, GLRO, HI/ST/NCI/72.
37. FN to J. Sutherland, GLRO, HI/ST/NCI/72, 6 January 1872.
40. Smith, B.F., *Florence Nightingale*, p. 163.
41. Donnison, *Midwives*, p. 81.
42. Cope, Z., *Florence Nightingale and the Doctors* (Methuen, London, 1958), p. 121.
43. Donnison, *Midwives*, p. 81.
44. H. Bonham Carter to FN, GLRO, HI/ST/SU/72/4, 24 May 1872.
45. FN to H. Acland, GLRO, HI/STN/CI/76, 1 January 1876, 6.30 a.m.
46. Ibid.
47. H. Bonham Carter to Geo. Frere, GLRO, HI/ST/NC18/12, 25 May 1876.
48. See Chapter 5.
49. Minutes, 2 March 1903. GLRO, A/NFC/2.2.

5. Poor Law Nursing

Before you decide what to do with the land [for building] would it not be better to decide what to do with the Poor Law which is rotten at the heart and wants cutting down to the root.

Florence Nightingale to William Rathbone, 1867

John Stuart Mill wrote that the 'principal business of the central authority should be to give instruction, the local authority to apply it. Power may be localised, but knowledge to be most useful must be centralised.'[1] In the matter of the Poor Law Miss Nightingale was a disciple of Mill and belonged to that group of radical liberals who believed that state intervention was the logical extension of the principles of Bentham. For this reason she was sometimes at odds with Poor Law reform groups who aimed at easing the lot of the sick pauper within the principles of the Poor Law Amendment Act of 1834.

If the subscribers to the Nightingale Fund had anything in mind it was no doubt the training of nurses in, and for, voluntary hospitals, but Miss Nightingale herself had always seen the need for trained nurses in Poor Law institutions. Since the inauguration of the Fund the problems of the sick in workhouses had grown worse, partly due to the effects of industrialisation and the vagaries of employment, but largely due to the 'workhouse test' and because the emphasis on indoor relief had exacerbated the vicious cycle of sickness and pauperism.

By the time the Nightingale training scheme was set up Poor Law reformers like Miss Louisa Twining with her Ladies Workhouse Visiting Association[2] and Dr Joseph Rogers of the Strand Union had uncovered a number of scandals and had revealed that over one-third of the workhouse inmates were sick; in the Metropolitan workhouses the figure for the adult able-bodied was as low as 10 per cent.[3] As early as 1856 Dr Rumsey had urged 'an administrative machine available for directing all measures for scientific relief of pauper sickness for maintaining public health, for investigating the prevalence of disease and mortality etc'.[4] Although every parish was different these reports and enquiries had revealed that medical and nursing coverage was totally inadequate and that in 1866 the 21,000 sick and aged in the London workhouses were cared for by only 142 paid, non-pauper, nurses.[5]

In Liverpool where the problem of pauperism could be seen at its worst[6] William Rathbone, the senior member of a firm of wealthy shipowners and a philanthropist in the Nonconformist tradition, turned his attention to the appalling conditions in the Brownlow Hill workhouse. The Vestry had made some effort to improve the conditions of the 1,000 sick paupers by employing a few paid nurses but these were untrained and had no authority over the pauper nurses.[7] Mr Rathbone, who had been in touch with Miss Nightingale in 1861 about a scheme for training district nurses, suggested to the Vestry that the key to improvement would be through the introduction of trained nurses. In 1864 he wrote to the Nightingale Fund offering to guarantee the cost if the Fund could supply a superintendent and a team of nurses. He also suggested that Miss Nightingale write to the governor, George Carr, without mentioning his name, because he wanted the governor 'who is a very clever man to have the kudos for the scheme.'[8]

Miss Nightingale and Dr Sutherland promised to think about the suggestion and Mr Rathbone accordingly made a submission to the Vestry saying that

> Justice and expediency alike counsel the introduction into the workhouse of the best system of nursing... the present system is failing for want of sufficient numbers of reliable and duly qualified nurses to carry out instructions given... [9]

From the first it seems that, in his enthusiasm, Rathbone made a deal with the Vestry before he was sure that the Fund could find a team and at the same time he inadvertently misled the Fund into thinking that the Vestry would meet all their conditions.

The problem for the Fund was to find a suitable superintendent. So far they had accepted 60 trainees of whom not more than 25 were still working so the choice was not wide. One possibility was Agnes Jones, the niece of Sir John Lawrence, the Viceroy of India, who was a friend of Miss Nightingale. Miss Jones had spent her childhood in India and seems to have had a history of mental depression; in adolescence she became intensely religious and this fervour was translated into a desire to nurse and to emulate Miss Nightingale. To this end she paid two visits to Kaiserwerth where in 1860, she was advised to undertake some hospital training. Miss Nightingale knew about Agnes Jones and was wary of accepting her. In a letter to Mary Jones she wrote:

> I cannot but think that her want of character is her peculiar character. She is always under someone's meridian. And you will see if she enters St Thomas's – which I am afraid she intends, she will write just such preaching letters to our old treasurer. Then there will be the same old story all over again.[10]

However, Mrs Wardroper was enthusiastic and Agnes was accepted and was a model pupil. Nevertheless there were worries about her health and at the end of the training while she was a sister at the Great Northern Hospital she was afflicted with 'nervous debility and deafness'; Mr Whitfield arranged for her to see Joseph Toynbee, the most eminent ear, nose and throat surgeon of his day who wrote that

> Miss Jones is suffering from partial nervous deafness in both ears, but not to such as extent as to be incapable of work. Cases of this kind are always exaggerated by ill health and are best treated by rest and fresh air... Objections to going to Liverpool would apply equally to undertaking any other nursing service. Let her go to Liverpool and enter on her nursing work. We cannot take into account anything that may happen afterwards... [11]

After many doubts Miss Jones felt that God had called her to Liverpool and Mr Whitfield sent her home to Ireland to recover. Miss Nightingale wrote to Mary Jones, 'Agnes Jones is in a fishing village in Ireland for her health, but I am so busy that I could have done without coping with the Liverpool experiment.'[12] This was an indication of both Miss Jones's health and Miss Nightingale's attitude to the problems of the Fund at that time: she was too busy with other things. There were then involved transactions with the Vestry. Mr Rathbone offered to pay for more accommodation at St Thomas's if more probationers could be sent to Liverpool,[13] but in the end all had to be kept at St Thomas's and paid for by Mr Rathbone because the agreement with the Vestry was not concluded and there was no accommodation for the nurses.

Miss Jones made a preliminary visit to Liverpool in August 1864 and took up her position in advance of the team in the spring. When the main party arrived on 16 May 1865, it was clear that in spite of the correspondence and Miss Jones's own negotiations the terms of reference were imprecise and the pauper nurses were still accountable to the governor. In July Miss Nightingale wrote inferring that the Fund had been deceived:

> The governors' intention all along had been to subordinate the nursing

to himself, just as if the superintendent and nurses were paupers. Now this cannot be, and after the facts have been discovered it must be dealt with. You cannot ask Mr Rathbone to spend £3,000 on the system Agnes Jones describes.[14]

There then followed what Dr Sutherland described as 'Hibernian rows' between the evangelical, Irish, Miss Jones and Mr Carr, but after visits to London and much pouring of oil on the troubled waters by Miss Nightingale, the situation settled into some sort of *modus vivendi*, and after two years the trained nurses were such a success – especially in the eyes of the Ladies Visiting Committee – that the Vestry was considering putting all the wards under their management.[15]

Back in London, and before the Liverpool scheme was even launched, Miss Nightingale had more pressing business relating to the Poor Law. On Christmas Eve 1864 there appeared in *The Times* a letter from James Shuter under the caption 'Horrible Case of Union Neglect' which referred to the death of Timothy Daly in the Holborn Workhouse. Miss Nightingale promptly wrote to Charles Villiers, the President of the Poor Law Board, and urged 'a searching enquiry into the whole question of workhouse nursing', adding that she would make an effort to see Mr Villiers on the subject.[16]

In January Mr Villiers duly came to South Street and Miss Nightingale adroitly used the Fund's co-operation with the Liverpool scheme as a model, though in fact the experiment had not started. Mr Villiers, aware of the precarious state of the Whig majority, was not prepared to apply compulsion to the Poor Law Board, but through Mr Villiers Miss Nightingale met Mr Farnall, the Poor Law inspector for the Metropolitan area, who wanted to take a more drastic line and who became Miss Nightingale's ally. It was through Mr Farnall that Miss Nightingale suggested that the Poor Law Board should seek information through a questionnaire and the form that was sent out with its 25 sections seems to bear her stamp.[17]

Meanwhile another pauper named Gibson died in February 1865 in St Giles's workhouse. *The Times* printed the inquest findings and led an attack on the whole Poor Law Medical Relief system. These and other revelations led James Wakley of *The Lancet* to set up *The Lancet Commission* which appointed three doctors, Ernest Hart of St Mary's, Dr Anstie of the Westminster and Dr Carr of Blackheath, to visit the metropolitan workhouses and to make reports. These were published in successive issues of *The Lancet*[18] from which we get a good picture of the conditions and the state of care for the 21,000 sick in the London workhouses at that time.

While Miss Nightingale kept up her pressure on Mr Villiers, other organisations fanned the flames. In February, at the instigation of Drs Rogers and Hart, The Association for Improving Workhouse Infirmaries was launched as a pressure group with a distinguished committee which included the Archbishop of York, the Earl of Carnarvon, Charles Dickens and John Stuart Mill. In a letter to her father Miss Nightingale inferred that she did not really approve because the Commission and the Association paid too little attention to nursing needs and did not get to the heart of the matter which was the Poor Law itself: 'It is *lèse-majesté* to ill use the imbecile woman, the dirty child – *philanthropy is the biggest humbug I know.* The principle must not be to punish the hungry for being hungry.'[19] However it is possible that she was in touch with the Association through Farnall and she sent her subscription. Moreover, the prospect of legislation caused the reformers to close their ranks. By May Miss Nightingale was identifying herself with the Association when she wrote to Harriet Martineau saying, 'We have been sending our Earls, Archbishops and M.P.s to storm him [Villiers] in his den'[20] and urged her to keep the pot boiling in the *Saturday Review.*[21]

As a result of this pressure Mr Villiers set up an enquiry and in July 1865 brought in an amended Bill which fell far short of the requirements of the reformers. In despair Miss Nightingale turned to the Prime Minister, Lord Palmerston, that old family friend whom she described as 'my most powerful protector'.[22]

Palmerston promised support in the next session and Miss Nightingale and Mr Farnall set about preparing a new draft. It is from one of these drafts that we get Miss Nightingale's 'A.B.C. Plan for Workhouse Reform' in which the sick were separated from the able-bodied and placed under one central management committee outside the Poor Law. In a draft she wrote:

> The sick and infirm require special constructive arrangements. They are not 'paupers', they are poor and in affliction. Society owes them every necessary care for their recovery... sickness is not parochial, it is general and should be borne by all.[23]

On 18 October 1865 Lord Palmerston died and the Whig government was tottering. In spite of the mounting campaign in the press and the medical journals and the evidence of overcrowding and neglect, Villiers remained cautious and little headway was made. Finally, on 18 June 1866, the government fell and with it the hopes of the reformers.

The new Tory administration under Lord Derby, now being educated by Disraeli in 'the art of dishing the Whigs', brought in their own legislation. This was cleverly contrived to silence popular clamour but conservative enough to satisfy their own ranks. Mr Villiers was replaced by Mr Gathorne Hardy to whom Miss Nightingale immediately wrote offering her services. Gathorne Hardy promptly set up a committee to report on the requisite space and other matters in relation to workhouse infirmaries with Sir Thomas Watson, the President of the Royal College of Physicians, as Chairman. It was a distinguished committee and included Captain Galton, the sanitary engineer and another Nightingale relative by marriage. Miss Nightingale was asked for suggestions[24] and her reply is contained in *Suggestions on the Subject of Providing Training and Organising Nurses for the Poor Sick in Workhouse Infirmaries.*[25] The covering letter begins with a typical Nightingale *bon mot*: 'I begin by taking it for granted that we mean the same thing by what is meant by the word nursing.' The 'Suggestions' were reprinted as a pamphlet and they follow closely the regulations, rules and conditions of training as those that were laid down for probationers under the Nightingale Fund, for Miss Nightingale always insisted that the principles of nursing and of training must be the same for the workhouse as for the general hospital.

However, when Mr Hardy drafted his Bill he largely ignored the advice of people like Chadwick, Mills, Rogers and Miss Nightingale who had advocated a central authority and went for a compromise which set up a new hospital authority for lunatics and fevers, but left the non-infectious poor sick under the Poor Law Boards in Unions. After reading Sir Harry Verney's advance copy of the bill Miss Nightingale wrote, 'The proposal to club five or six Unions together for the sick is absurd – the little that has leaked out suggests the Bill will be a failure.[26] Sir Harry, and other Fund Council members who were Members of Parliament were urged to press for amendments and Sir Harry succeeded in getting inserted a clause that the new hospitals should be used for training nurses.[27]

Writing to the Association for the Improvement of Workhouse Infirmaries, Miss Nightingale set out the defects of the Bill in pungent language – worth recording because it embodies her concept of good administration and is why she kept the Fund Council small and did not waste its time with sub-committees:

> Good administration is not provided by the Bill. What is contemplated is to continue under certain improved conditions the same sort of thing that has existed but with a better system of inspection in the hope that evil will be prevented. But this is the very principle of administration to be avoided. Inspection involved the idea of lax administration and failure to be remedied by punishing someone for neglect of duty. This is fatal. The real principle should be to provide Central Management for the whole Metropolis. All hospitals should be managed by paid, responsible

officers under conditions planned to ensure success. The head of the administration should be a first rate business man... no hospital committees of management are required... the only committee required is a financial one.[28]

The Metropolitan Poor Act became law on 29 March 1867 and the following year the Poor Law Amendment Act gave similar powers to provincial authorities. One of the main objectives was to produce much needed separate accommodation for fever cases and lunatics. To achieve this a Metropolitan Asylums Board was set up with the power to build and run such hospitals from a Common Fund; this produced no hostility from the upholders of the less eligibility principle, because it was unlikely that paupers would go either into a fever hospital or a lunatic asylum to get preferential treatment. The problem of the non-infectious sick was different. If the sick and infirm were removed the Guardians would have been left with only 11 per cent of their inmates and less eligibility would have been in shreds.[29] Therefore the Act set up Sick Asylums Districts and Poor Law Unions were reorganised and encouraged to build separate infirmaries for non-infectious cases. The new Act did not use compulsion, but, by using the carrot and stick of the Common Fund, Poor Law Unions were penalised if they did not comply because they then had to provide the salaries of doctors and nurses out of their own poor rate. However, the value of the carrot was soon seen to be illusory because building costs rose and capital outlay outweighed the advantages the Common Fund bestowed on running costs. The hospital building programme proved more costly than anticipated.

One of the first Unions to take advantage of the Bill was St Pancras. The St Pancras Union had been through many vicissitudes; censured by Dr Bence Jones in 1854, who was now a member of the Fund Council, it had improved and had been partly rebuilt and now had 16 paid non-pauper nurses.[30] However, it had recently been censured by the coroner about a case of a child prematurely laid out 'and treated as dead before she had wholly expired because there were not sufficient numbers of paid medical attendants and nurses to perform the duties of so large an establishment'.[31] Now, led by the chairman of the Reform Group, Mr Wyatt, the Guardians decided to build a new infirmary in Upper Holloway, Highgate (which later became the Whittington Hospital), and, duly advised by Mr Wyatt, they appealed to the Nightingale Fund for help in providing nursing staff for part of the new hospital. As it happened Mr Gathorne Hardy's reign at the Poor Law Board was short and with his departure policy about new buildings changed. However, the St Pancras

Guardians were allowed to continue with their plans and when finished the infirmary was transferred to the Central London Sick Asylum. These changes in control account for some of the difficulties faced by the Fund in setting up the nursing scheme at Highgate. To complicate matters in 1871, as the scheme was being set up, the old Poor Law Board with whom the Fund was used to negotiating was replaced by a new Local Government Board.

While the preliminary discussions were going on with Mr Wyatt and the St Pancras Guardians, disaster struck at the Fund's other Poor Law nursing scheme in Liverpool. Agnes Jones, who was said to be working from 5.30 a.m. to 1.30 a.m. caught typhus and eventually died on 19 February 1868. A highly wrought and sentimental account of the last two weeks of Agnes' illness is provided in the almost daily letters from Miss Elizabeth Gilpin, a lady visitor, to Miss Nightingale, ending with 'our darling is at rest'.[32] Agnes Jones's two aunts, Georgina and Esther Smythe (who had come to Liverpool to be with her at the end and stayed for three months to run the nursing) were described by Miss Nightingale as 'two very unwise but excellent old ladies'. Agnes, it seems was incapable of delegating and now there was no one to take over.

Mrs Wardroper, urged on by Mr Rathbone, looked for a successor and sent Louise Freeman who had only done four months' training, and who, it was alleged, 'treated the Probationers like reformed convicts'. Miss Freeman soon resigned and was replace by Miss Lucy Kidd, a Special who Mrs Wardroper recorded as having 'an exemplary character'. Admirers of the saintly Miss Jones predicted failure, and not apparently without reason, for Miss Kidd was dismissed by the Vestry because of her intoxication.

Meanwhile Miss Nightingale, trying to save something from the wreck, published her article 'Una and the Lion' in *Good Words*. This was a thinly disguised eulogy of Agnes Jones, but after a sentimental and contrived opening, she stepped adroitly aside into a straightforward, hard-hitting appeal for women, of any class, to come forward and train as hospital nurses; this was in fact blatant advertising for the Fund with details for application set out at the bottom, and it contains some of Miss Nightingale's most pungent writing on the subject. In the final paragraphs she returns to 'Una' and her funeral with the devoted village children dropping primroses and violets and weeping over the grave.

Presumably this was not enough for the Jones family and a sister of Agnes insisted on writing a Memorial.[33] This caused Miss Nightingale to write in alarm saying that such a publication would have a disastrous effect on the cause of workhouse nursing: 'It was workhouse nursing that made and brought her out of this insufferable family twaddle.'[34] It is doubtful if the Memorial, when it came, was widely read enough to do harm but in it the sister makes the claim that 'Agnes carried out real Bible work in her hospital work and sought to lead sinners to repentance[35] – a statement which would have filled Guardians, who dreaded competing sectarian proselytising, with horror. Miss Nightingale had some grounds for concern. Later she complained of getting 'long and vulgar' letters from Miss Gilpin and fussy maundering accounts from the aunts with stories of miracles related by Agnes, which made her write that this 'painfully convinces me of the truth of what I have been told about Agnes, that her mind was going some months before her death owing to continual deficient sleep and her naturally anxious disposition'.[36]

Since the story of Agnes Jones is so overlaid with myth it is probable that the truth will never be known. It seems likely that she was an immature personality with a tendency to depressive phases and given to intense friendships which she often inspired in others. Nevertheless, fortified with a devout faith, when the challenge came she overcame her diffidence and her Irish temper.

Miss Nightingale was probably right when she said 'Workhouse nursing made her'; when she was too busy and tired to be anxious about her spiritual health she coped, but the fact that the experiment more or less collapsed with her death shows that she had laid no permanent foundation. Her family, who were much concerned with her memory, would have surely been gratified that she was eventually commemorated in stained glass.

Whatever 'Una and the Lion' did for recruitment in London it did nothing for Liverpool. The dismissal of Miss Kidd was humiliating and the Vestry was no longer interested in the experiment. In 1870 a disillusioned Miss Nightingale wrote to Sir John McNeill:

> they have not now got one woman left in our training school. They have got rid of all our nurses not because they deserve to be dismissed but because they deserve promotion. Some we have taken back, one has gone as a nurse to Agnes Jones' mother and three as sisters to the Middlesex.[37]

Miss Nightingale did not add that of the team sent from St Thomas's Agnes Jones herself had dismissed three. The three that were sent to the Middlesex can be found in the Middlesex records and their fate casts some reflection on Miss Nightingale's opinion that the Nightingale team 'deserved promotion'. Miss Thorold, the new matron of the Middlesex, dismissed Maria Trueman as 'being unfit for the post of sister'; Elizabeth Harvey was dismissed because of 'an ungovernable temper and want of subordination'. However, the third, Elizabeth

Trueman, was said to be 'a conscientious woman and an excellent head nurse'.[38]

As usual Mr Rathbone tried to salvage the situation by offering more money, but Miss Nightingale wrote:

> I am anxious to do what we can for Mr Rathbone, but we must not let him get the bit between his teeth and spoil other work... one cannot look upon Liverpool as much of a success. I believe the difficulties have been brought about by attempting too much and not starting on a sound basis.[39]

Later, after the dismissal of Miss Kidd and further difficulties with the Vestry, Mr Bonham Carter wrote:

> The proposal [to continue] cannot be entertained. Unless we enter the new building [at St Thomas's] with an efficient staff our training will fare badly, the organisation at Liverpool is such that we could not send a superintendent.[40]

Mr Bonham Carter might have added that the Fund had not got a superintendent to send. One reason for the failure of the Liverpool scheme was that either Miss Jones had no one of the calibre to train as deputy, or that she was incapable of delegation, and on her death the Fund had no one as her replacement. The Fund had attempted much, but after ten years it realised that it was 'not starting on a sound basis'.

Back in London negotiations were going on between the Fund and Mr Wyatt of the St Pancras Guardians about the possibility of finding a superintendent for the new Highgate Infirmary. The choice fell on Elizabeth Torrance, a Scotch Presbyterian who was one of the first Special Probationers, and who in December 1868, accompanied by Mrs Wardroper, went to inspect the new 500-bed hospital and to meet the Guardians. Both ladies 'pronounced satisfaction at what they saw'.

Although the Fund Council was aware that the new hospital opened possibilities for introducing reformed nursing into the Poor Law on the lines laid down in Miss Nightingale's paper, there were difficulties. The Fund was short of people of superintendent calibre and there were not likely to be many occasions where people as outstanding as Mr Wyatt and Miss Torrance came together. Second, there was the question of finance. In his *Notes on Establishing a Good Training School for Workhouse Nurses*, Mr Bonham Carter set out the advantages and disadvantages of training becoming a government responsibility. He suggested that at Highgate the Fund 'may do more successfully if it spends some capital', and he points out that experience had shown that the Boards of Guardians would not pay for train-

ing but above all the probationers must not be selected by the
Guardians but solely by the Principal of the training school.[41] On the
other hand, Mr Bonham Carter noted, if the Fund spent money they
were merely saving the hospital money and he reiterated that at
St Thomas's the number of staff were diminished as a consequence of
the use made of the Fund's probationers.

Eventually, after many delays, Miss Torrance and nine nurses,
some of whom had not finished their training year, took up residence
at Highgate. Miss Torrance saw that the only way to overcome the
problem of pauper nurses was to train her own and by the end of 1870
Mr Bonham Carter, having talked the matter over with Mr Wyatt,
wrote to Miss Nightingale: 'I propose to spend a limited amount of
money on making a commencement of a training school, £100-£120
– say six probationers at £60, £24 for clothes and £52 for gratuities.'
This item does not appear in the Committee's minutes until the
following year so it must be assumed that Mr Bonham Carter took the
decision himself, or more likely discussed it informally with other
committee members, probably Sir John Clark who usually audited the
accounts and who was related by marriage. Although Mr Wyatt was
able to get permission for the training school for the Central London
Sick Asylums District, Mr Bonham Carter expressed a doubt about
the legality of the matron having power to select and dismiss probationers without reference to the authority – a doubt that was to prove
justified later. However, and presumably as a result of the Highgate
experiment, in 1873 the Central London Sick Asylum District was
authorised under Section 29 of the Act to 'receive single women or
widows between the ages of 25 and 35 years as probationers... under
the control of the medical officer and the matron'.

The training arrangements between the Fund and the Board of
Guardians were similar to those at St Thomas's except that Miss
Torrance and Dr Dowse, the medical officer who eventually agreed to
help with the training, were paid less, and Miss Torrance insisted on
dropping the phrase in the regulations that 'probationers would receive
instruction from head nurses' because her head nurses were not
capable of giving instruction. Miss Nightingale, in requesting
Mr Bonham Carter to make the amendment, goes on to say, 'It has been
a universal and increasing complaint among our good probationers that
our sisters do not give the instructions promised in the regulations.'[42]

Miss Nightingale liked Miss Torrance and kept in touch with her
and, in view of her later attitude to her favourites who married, one
comment is interesting:

> Miss Torrance's influence depends on her excessive interest in her
> nurses as individuals. She is the only person I have ever heard say

cordially 'You know I like the women to marry – I think that class are happier when married'.[43]

Miss Torrance's competence and interest in her nurses seems borne out in the fact that the nurses who went with her stayed, most remaining to collect their last gratuity. The probationers had a reasonably good success rate and the Central District Board was pleased with the scheme. Unfortunately Miss Torrance was transferred back to St Thomas's in 1872 and there was much heart searching for a suitable successor. The choice eventually fell on Annie Hill, a free Special who, although she had been a governess to her cousin Shore's children, was unknown to Miss Nightingale. Miss Hill did not have the same support as did Miss Torrance and the relationship between her and Mrs Wardroper seems to have soured. Mrs Wardroper resented the fact that Miss Torrance had been brought back as a watchdog, and it appears as if this spilled over into a resentment against the whole Highgate set up, and Dr Dowse, whom Miss Torrance was eventually to marry.[44]

Nevertheless, Miss Hill proved capable of standing her ground and her reports are clear and legible. In 1873 she had a brisk correspondence with Mr Bonham Carter because Mr Appleton, the Clerk to the Board, insisted on paying the probationers himself, and she wrote that the nurses came from a class where they equated the person who paid them with the person who had the power to dismiss them, and she asks if anything can be done to overturn the rule.[45] It seems that the new Local Government Board did not like any staff being under the control of anyone but themselves. Mr Bonham Carter did intervene and Miss Hill at least retained a semblance of control, an episode which illustrates that the main battle about getting trained nurses into Poor Law institutions was not so much the principle of training but the problem of accountability.

The work at Highgate increased rapidly. Miss Torrance had warned that the nursing was heavier than at St Thomas's and the sick were now being admitted direct from home. Miss Hill, who had nine nurses and six probationers and pauper nurses, was clearly overworked. Miss Nightingale, once she started seeing Miss Hill, took a more sympathetic view:

> Miss Hill is in a state where she cannot go on without serious injury to herself and the work. (She has promised to go to Embley this day week.) She tells me 'my headaches are almost more than I can bear'.[46]

Mr Bonham Carter replied by sending his wife Sibella to ascertain what state Miss Hill was in[47] and she took a less dramatic view of the situation. However, as Miss Hill was to die in 1877 of what seems to have been a long terminal illness, it is possible that her headaches were preludes to more sinister symptoms.

Nevertheless, in spite of Mrs Wardroper's scathing remarks and Miss Nightingale's damning with faint praise, 'killing herself with conscientiousness and unbusiness-like-ness – but we have no one with a higher moral tone than she has',[48] Miss Hill managed to keep her staff together, the approbation of Dr Dowse, and her assistant Sarah Hinks who, while Miss Hill lay dying, seems to have acted with spirit and common sense. It was thought that Miss Hinks would take over, but at the age of 46 the Local Government Board ruled that she was too old. Once again the Fund had no one suitable to send, but the following month Mrs Wardroper suggested a Miss Luckling[49] who had been admitted as a Special to train for the Metropolitan and National Nursing Association. Miss Luckling was duly appointed as matron, but after two months she was dismissed by the Board for inefficiency. Miss Hinks resigned two months later and, as the Board proposed a matron not of the Fund's choosing, after consulting with Miss Nightingale Mr Bonham Carter withdrew the Fund's nurses.[50] Miss Hinks made a careful inventory of the equipment and books given as a bequest to the School and, after some difficulty, ensured their return to St Thomas's.

The Fund report of 1877 stated that

Only part of the original object for which the school was established was attained, for in consequence of the small number of probationers the supply of trained nurses was exhausted by the requirements of the Infirmary itself and no other Infirmary has derived benefit from the School.[51]

In other words the Highgate scheme had no missionary value. However, as the Fund did not expend capital and only set aside £200 a year for the School, to expect the experiment to staff the growing needs of the Highgate Infirmary and to act as a missionary force was perhaps a little ambitious. The real reason for the withdrawal was undoubtedly the fact that the Fund had not got a superintendent acceptable to the Guardians and they would not leave Nightingale nurses accountable to anyone but a trained nurse of whom they approved.

Apart from the failure to find enough money to finance the scheme or enough suitable probationers and training sisters, another reason for the apparent failure of the scheme was the changed attitude of the Local Government Board. Faced with the economic depression of the 1870s and the criticism of the old guard, the high hopes of the even limited reforms of Gathorne Hardy died away. Miss Nightingale wrote bitterly of the new 'Sick Asylums': 'I do not believe that they are an improvement on the old workhouse infirmaries – the P.L.B. interferes about trifles and inspection is useless. Sic Transit *ingloria* Mundi without offering any reform.'[52]

The closure of the school at Highgate seems symptomatic of the weakness of the Metropolitan Poor Law Act and it indicates that the reformers' demands for a Central Fund and a measure of compulsion were justified. By 1873 nine separate infirmaries had been opened in London but the system of employing pauper nurses had not been superseded and there were six Unions without any special institution for the sick.[53] Moreover, although the Central London Sick Asylums District was allowed to train nurses, since few authorities employed trained nurses this authority was largely illusory. In 1879 this failure to provide better nursing led Miss Twining's ladies to form The Association for Promoting Trained Nursing in Workhouse Asylums with William Bowman, a Fund Council member, on the Central Committee. Although Miss Nightingale did not always see eye to eye with Miss Twining there was much in the Association's aims with which she must have agreed, and Miss Nightingale's red pencil seems to have descended but once on the report of the inaugural meeting and that on the statement that 'the same amount of skilled training was not needed for all nurses [in infirmaries] as in general hospitals'. The report gives some interesting facts: when, for example, the 1861 census gave a figure of 10,414 for inmates of voluntary hospitals there were 80,000 sick persons in workhouses and, in an anecdote, it gives the unwitting testimony that the 'town' hospitals were passing on their 'incurables' to the Poor Law infirmaries.[54]

Miss Twining wrote to Miss Nightingale to ask if anything was being done by the Fund to assist with the training of nurses for Workhouse infirmaries.[55] The reply is not available but shortly afterwards the Fund was approached by Mr Boulnois, the chairman of the St Marylebone Guardians, who explained that they were building a new infirmary in Ladbroke Grove – later known as St Charles's Hospital – and the committee were considering the arrangements for nursing for which they asked for help and advice. The Fund Committee considered the request as its meeting on 10 May 1881 and agreed to supply a superintendent and a team of nurses, and to contribute to the expenses of a training school under similar conditions to those adopted in the arrangements with Highgate, the contributions not to exceed £200 a year.

After much consultation the choice for a superintendent fell on Elizabeth Vincent, one of the group of Specials who trained in 1872 and who probably owe their success to the fact that there were enough of them to support one another. Miss Vincent did not apparently impress Mrs Wardroper, but Miss Nightingale called her a 'fine fellow – as true as steel'. After a spell at Lincoln as matron she returned home to look after a sick father. Her return to the service of the Fund as Miss Machin's assistant at St Bartholomew's was not a happy episode, but Miss Machin was equally unsettled. Miss Vincent wanted the post at St Marylebone and she was lucky inasmuch as Dr Lunn from St Thomas's was appointed as Resident Medical Officer at the same time. This encouraged Miss Nightingale to write to Mr Bonham Carter, 'when you think of putting in a small training school there will be advantages that she, and almost all her staff, are accustomed to training'.

Before the team of nine left there was a lengthy correspondence between Mr Boulnois and Mr Bonham Carter about plans for the new Nurses' Home with Miss Nightingale insisting on more bathrooms, better ventilation and a sick room. On the question of a nurse training school Mr Boulnois pointed out that the Local Government Board would not authorise expenditure on nurses not required in running the hospital and he asked the Fund to assist. The Fund agreed to pay the cost of probationers 'reasonably required' but would not bind themselves to a specific period. Mr Bonham Carter suggested that the government should pay towards adapting the new building as a School of Nursing which would have as its aim the 'supply of trained nurses for other Poor Law infirmaries in London'. There is no evidence that the Board did pay.

In due course a five-year contract was signed with the Fund[56] requiring that each probationer be supplied with board, lodging, washing and uniform, and be under the authority of the matron.

As at St Thomas's the probationers were to serve as assistant nurses on the wards, to have instruction from head nurses and to receive class teaching from medical officers. Then came the stumbling block: 'that probationers be selected by the matron and would be subject to be dismissed by her and that they should be bound to the Fund to enter into service as infirmary nurses... the St Marylebone Board of Guardians having a preferential claim'. In September 1882 Mr Rotton, a clerk to the Local Government Board, wrote that the Board had directed him to point out

> that the arrangements which were approved by them with regard to probationer nurses in the sick asylums were made under the 30th Victoria Cap. 6 Section 29, which provides that an asylum is provided under the Act for the reception and relief of the Sick Poor may be used for training of nurses in such cases and in such a manner and subject to

the Regulations as the Local Government Board direct. The enactment
does not apply to the Parish of St. Marylebone and the arrangements
suggested cannot legally be carried out...[57]

Joseph Bedord, clerk to the Board of Guardians, suggested that a way
round the problem would be for the Board to 'elect' the persons
recommended by the Fund and urged the Local Government to
approve 12 probationers.[58] The Board refused to sanction more than
eight and Mr Bonham Carter stood firm and refused to ratify the
agreement. This brought a visit from Mr Boulnois and a compromise
was worked out with the Fund agreeing to waive rule six that 'probationers will be required to enter into hospitals service in such situations
that may from time to time be offered by the Committee'.[59]

When the alterations to the Home were made, and after considerable correspondence, Miss Vincent, two head nurses and seven ward
nurses took up their post in the new 760-bedded hospital. There was
some delay in finding a Home sister but in 1883 Gertrude Wyld took
up her post as training sister which she held until 1887 when she was
replaced by Miss Moriarty who did much, in harness with Dr Lunn,
to make the school such a success. In 1883 the school received prestige and publicity when the Home was opened by HRH Princess
Christian, possibly the first time that royalty had graced a Poor Law
institution. By 1885 there were 12 probationers and already there were
six who had trained in the school on the staff. In the next 20 years
there continued to be a considerable exchange of nursing staff between
St Thomas's and St Marylebone, the latter providing a useful stepping
stone for wider experience.

During this period the Fund Council displayed great interest in
workhouse infirmaries. In 1878 Sir William Wyatt came on to the
Fund Council and in 1889 he was joined by Edmund Boulnois MP,
two men with long experience in the battle for workhouse infirmary
reform. In 1883 the Fund sent matron, Miss Styring, an assistant
matron, the night sister and two head nurses to the Paddington New
Parochial Infirmary, whose staff was in time supplemented from
St Marylebone, and which, in due course, opened its own training
school. Amy Hughes, later well known as the director of the Queen's
Jubilee nurses, became the matron of the Bolton Infirmary and other
trainees went to other infirmaries. Nightingale nurses eventually
returned to Brownlow Hill in Liverpool and supplied much of its staff.

When Miss Vincent retired in 1899 she was admitting 20–30
probationers a year, the school was offering a wide range of lectures
and the successful candidates were going out to nursing posts all over
the country; many were becoming head nurses in other infirmaries so

the report of 1899 stated:

> The Committee wish to place on record their high appreciation of the
> valuable service Miss Vincent has rendered to the cause of nursing, not
> only as head of the nursing staff at the Infirmary but also as contributing
> to that influence for good which the infirmary has undoubtedly exercised
> to similar institutions.[60]

Miss Vincent was succeeded by Miss Lucy Ramsden, a trainee of
St Thomas's who unfortunately retired within three years on grounds
of ill health. At this point the Fund decided to sever its connection with
the school, not from any dissatisfaction, but because of economic pressure, and because it was assured that the foundations were well laid
and that the school could carry on without the Fund. This hope was
apparently realised because in 1909 there is a letter from Miss
Cockerell, the matron, inviting Mr Bonham Carter, who was then over
80 years old, to come and see the school and the newly furnished
wards. The informal connection remained for some time and the
St Marylebone School of Nursing must be counted as one of the
Fund's most successful ventures.

It is arguable that the Fund's influence on nursing in workhouse
infirmaries in the period 1880 to 1900 was greater than its influence
on nursing in general hospitals. With the advancement of medical
science and the general movement for useful and remunerative
employment for middle-class women, training schools would have
developed without the influence of the Fund. Indeed, many did and,
as Miss Nightingale herself said, many hospitals 'had as good or better
trainings'. The breakthrough in workhouse nursing was more difficult
largely because of the attitude of the Local Government Board that all
staff must be accountable to the Guardians. Had not the Fund been
persistent and cut through the Gordian knot it is possible that a trained
nursing service would have been longer delayed in infirmaries and that
the new municipal hospitals would have been considered even more
'second class' than they were. The poor sick owe much to pioneers like
Agnes Jones, Elizabeth Torrance, Annie Hill and Elizabeth Vincent.

Notes

1. Mill, J.S., *Considerations of Representative Government* (London, 1866),
   1912 edn., p. 376.
2. Abel Smith, B., *A History of the Nursing Profession* (Heinemann, London,
   1960), p. 37f.
3. Hodgkinson, R.G., *The Origins of the National Health Service* (Wellcome,
   London, 1867), p. 466.

4. Rumsey, H.W., *Essays in State Medicine*, quoted in Hodgkinson, p. 464.
5. Smith, E., *Report on Metropolitan Infirmaries from M.O. to the Poor Law Board*, BPP 1867–8, vol. x, House of Commons 4, 6/24.
6. Chadwick, E., *The Sanitary Condition of the Labouring Population of Great Britain* (reprinted with an introduction by M.W. Flinn, 1965). See 'Comparative Chances of Life in Different Classes in the Community', Document 3a in Fraser, D., *The Evolution of the British Welfare State* (Macmillan, London, 1973), p. 240.
7. Liverpool refused to implement the Poor Law Amendment Act and there had been a special Liverpool Act to allow it to retain its former administration – the Vestries.
8. W. Rathbone to H. Bonham Carter, GLRO, HI/ST/NC18.4(12), 2 July 1864.
9. Hardy, G., *William Rathbone and Early District Nursing* (Hesketh, London, 1983), quoting the Submission to the Select Vestry, June 1864.
10. FN to Mary Jones, GLRO, HI/ST/NC1/61.3, 25 May 1861.
11. J. Toynbee to J. Sutherland, BL, Add Mss 45751, 30 June 1864, f. 239.
12. FN to Mary Jones, GLRO, HI/ST/NC1/64, 16 July 1864.
13. Wardroper to H. Bonham Carter; Baggally to H. Bonham Carter, GLRO, HI/ST/NC18/4, 13, 14 & 18 July 1864.
14. FN to J. Bonham Carter, BL, Add Mss 45752, 13 August 1865, f. 51.
15. E. Gilpin to FN, BL, Add Mss 45800, 8 February 1862, f. 220.
16. FN to C.P. Villiers (draft), BL, Add Mss 45789, December 1864, f. 54.
17. Copy of printed questionnaire to Poor Law authorities. BL, Add Mss 45792, May 1865, f. 14.
18. Hodgkinson, *Origins*, p. 472.
19. FN to W.E. Nightingale, BL, Add Mss 45790, 12 October 1865, f. 352.
20. Ayers, G., *England's First State Hospitals* (Wellcome, London, 1971), p. 9. See also Cook, *Florence Nightingale*, vol. 2, p. 105.
21. FN to H. Martineau, BL, Add Mss 45792, February 1865, f. 280.
22. Ridley, J., *Lord Palmerston* (Constable, London, 1970), p. 584.
23. Undated draft for Dr Sutherland, BL, Add Mss 45792, f. 32. See also Ayers, *England's First State Hospitals*, p. 8. and Woodham-Smith, Florence Nightingale, p. 467.
24. Thos. Watson to FN, BL, Add Mss 45800, 5 January 1867, f. 24.
25. 'Suggestions on the Subject of Providing Training and Organising nurses for the Poor Sick in Workhouses', 19 January 1867, contained in government report (no. xvi, pp. 64–79), *To Consider the Cubic Space in Metropolitan Workhouse Infirmaries*.
26. FN to Sir H. Verney, *Claydon Papers*, 1 March 1867.
27. Ayers, *England's First State Hospitals*, pp. 23–4.
28. FN to J. Parkinson, BL, Add Mss 45800, 7 February 1867, f. 54.
29. Ayers, *England's First State Hospitals*, pp. 23–4.
30. Hodgkinson, *Origins*, p. 455.
31. *The Lancet*, 31 June 1866, p. 354.
32. E. Gilpin to FN, BL, Add Mss 45800, 19 February 1868, f. 247.

33. Jones A., *Agnes Jones – A Memorial by her Sister* (Strachan, London, 1869).

34. FN to W. Rathbone, BL Add Mss 47754, January 1869, f. 215.

35. Jones – Agnes Jones's Sister.

36. FN to W. Rathbone, BL, Add Mss 47754, 29 January 1869, f. 221.

37. FN to Sir J. McNeill, GLRO, HI/ST/NC3SU161, 8 February 1870.

38. *The Middlesex Hospital Record Office Register of Sisters and Nurses, 1869–1873.*

39. FN to H. Bonham Carter, BL, Add Mss 47715, 2 March 1868, f. 192.

40. H. Bonham Carter to Sir J. McNeill, GLRO, HI/ST/NC18,11(1), 10 October 1870.

41. H. Bonham Carter to FN, GLRO, HI/ST/NC2/V22.71, 25 June 1871.

42. FN to H. Bonham Carter, BL, Add Mss 47717, 24 November 1871, ff. 8–9.

43. FN to H. Bonham Carter, BL, Add Mss 47717, 24 November 1871, f. 10.

44. See Chapter 9.

45. A. Hill to H. Bonham Carter, GLRO, HI/ST/NC18.11 (9, 7, 10), 25 November 1873.

46. FN to H. Bonham Carter, BL, Add Mss 47719, 30 June 1874, f. 49.

47. H. Bonham Carter to FN, BL, Add Mss 47719, July 1874, f. 51.

48. FN to H. Bonham Carter, BL, Add Mss 45800, 1 October 1874, f. 21.

49. H. Bonham Carter to FN, GLRO, HI/ST/NC18.13(19), 11 September 1877.

50. H. Bonham Carter to Sir. H. Verney, ibid., 23 and 24 December 1877.

51. *Nightingale Fund Council Report,* 1877.

52. FN to H. Bonham Carter, BL, Add Mss 47717, f. 24 (n.d.).

53. Abel-Smith, B., *The Hospitals* (Heinemann, London, 1964), pp. 94 and 98.

54. Printed report of the inaugural meeting of the Association for Promoting Trained Nursing in Workhouse Infirmaries. GLRO, HI/ST/NC15, 13d, July 1979.

55. L. Twining to FN, GLRO, HI/ST/NC18.26, 1880.

56. The 1982 Agreement with St Marylebone Infirmary, GLRO, HI/ST/NC18.31(7).

57. J. Bedford to H. Bonham Carter, GLRO, HI/ST/NC18.31.

58. H. Bonham Carter to J. Bedford, ibid., 30 October 1882.

59. E. Boulnois to H. Bonham Carter, BL, Add Mss 47729, 21 December 1882, f. 242.

60. *The Nightingale Fund Council Report,* 1899.

6. Nursing in Military Hospitals

The experience of the Military Hospitals in the East led to the introduction through Miss Nightingale's advice and influence of a permanent addition of Female Nurses as part of the regular staff of the British Army, and a beginning was made at Netley and Chatham Hospitals with a small staff of superintendents and nurses from the School at St Thomas's Hospital.

Report of the Nightingale Fund Council, 1910

When Miss Nightingale discussed taking a group of nurses to Scutari with Lord Palmerston, it is said that Lady Palmerston was taken aback because she recalled that in the Peninsular War army 'nurses' were camp followers of doubtful repute.[1] In spite of conflicts and disputes, one thing Miss Nightingale's somewhat mixed band of nurses did establish was that female nurses, properly trained, disciplined and employed, could be an asset to the Army Medical Service.

On her return to England Miss Nightingale's first priorities were the reform of the Army Medical Services and to ensure that there was a proper training establishment for army doctors with research and statistical collecting facilities. Allied to this was the need to persuade the War Office to accept a cadre of trained nurses as part of the staff of permanent peacetime military hospitals. In order for such a service to function properly it was necessary that there should be at least two military hospitals built according to the most modern, hygienic and labour-saving plans. These objectives were embodied in the findings of the Royal Commission which had four sub-committees. They are the objectives set out in Miss Nightingale's own evidence, which was the basis of much of the Commission's final report.

While the Commission was sitting, plans for a new army hospital at Southampton Water were underway. Miss Nightingale disapproved of the plan and the site. The plan for Netley was based on long corridor lines, and she was now pioneering the pavilion plan and using Lariboisière as a model, but Lord Panmure, the Secretary of State for

War, declared that at this stage the plans could not be changed. That Christmas Miss Nightingale happened to spend a night at Broadlands, and she appealed to the Prime Minister, Lord Palmerston, who was convinced that Miss Nightingale was right and who sent a strongly worded note to Lord Panmure. However, Lord Panmure feared the wrath of the Treasury and trouble in his own department, and in spite of articles in *The Builder*,[2] except for minor modifications, the plans remained unchanged. Ridley writes that 'for over a hundred years people connected with Netley agree that Miss Nightingale was right',[3] a statement that is vindicated by the fact that the hospital was demolished in 1966. The plan for Netley is important because when the Fund was asked to supply nurses much of the vast correspondence between the Fund and the War Office relates to adapting the building and finding suitable quarters for the nurses.

During the discussions on the plan for Netley Lord Panmure asked Miss Nightingale for a confidential report on Female Nursing in Military Hospitals. This report – duly expanded – was printed as *Subsidiary Notes on the Introduction of Female Nursing into Military Hospitals in War and Peace*[4] and contains Miss Nightingale's ideas on nursing in general as they had developed by 1858, and the *Notes* form the basis for the regulations and conditions laid down by the Fund for its Schools. *Subsidiary Notes* show Miss Nightingale's vast knowledge of both hospitals in England and in Europe and the different systems of providing care at that date; her recommendations are the result of reflection on the merits and demerits of the different systems and plans. However, throughout the *Notes* Miss Nightingale insists that progress must be slow and in the early stages there must be room for change 'unfettered by rules'. That said, she makes a number of detailed recommendations for the organisation of both civil and military nursing, some of which became standard practice for the next hundred years. The ward routine, including the times for sweeping and cleaning, bedmaking and the doctor's rounds, the patient/staff ratio, the ward linen service, who should do what, when and where, it is all there. Mercifully, Miss Nightingale was adamant about the importance of labour-saving devices, and no one can say that domestic cleaning was part of the Nightingale tradition. But there was a heavy emphasis on 'duty' and the necessity of the head nurse being on call to her patients day and night with her bed-sitting room off the ward and there are literally pages devoted to how these rooms should be furnished, even to the best way of finding a labour-saving substitute for black-leading grates. No detail is too small.

Running through the *Notes* there is the conviction that hospitals, both military and civil, were corrupting and even dangerous places and the less chance there was of young women gossiping in corridors or being molested on the stairs the better. On the subject of choosing female nursing staff for military hospitals Miss Nightingale agreed that it was right, other things being equal, to give preference to army surgeons' and officers' widows, but with the warning that 'misconduct in women is more pernicious in a military hospital than any other'. To minimise the chance she advocated that there should be as few women as possible, that a nursing sister should never do what can be done by an orderly and only those of head nurse calibre should be employed; they should be 'given responsibility and plenty to do',[5] and should not normally be recruited under the age of 30 years.

Even when the alterations were complete Netley was a disappointment: 'It is behind the day. It is not such a hospital as the great Military Hospital of the Empire should be. It would make a model barracks for 2,000 men.'[6] It was one of the longest hospitals in the world, 468 yards long rising above, and reflected in, Southampton Water. The hospital was eventually completed in 1862 with Mrs Jane Shaw Stewart as the superintendent. Mrs Shaw Stewart had gone to the Crimea with Mary Stanley's party. An experienced nurse, she knew most of the hospitals in Europe and was, like Miss Nightingale herself, patrician in outlook, well connected, her brother Michael, for example, being a Member of Parliament. Through the family's High Church connections she was also friendly with the Herberts and in fact Sidney Herbert's last letter was addressed to her. In the Crimea Miss Nightingale had found her a hard worker and a 'true heroine'[7] and when she thought she was dying, Miss Nightingale, in her 'Last Letter' to Sidney Herbert, commended Jane Shaw Stewart as superintendent of Netley. On her return from the Crimea Mrs Shaw Stewart sent long letters to Miss Nightingale; she disliked the idea of the Fund and thought it would be a hindrance to the cause of nursing, but she continued to send Miss Nightingale advice about possible hospitals as training schools.[8] In the meantime she spent some time at St Thomas's as a pupil of Mr Whitfield studying surgical nursing, from where she sent Miss Nightingale long accounts.

In 1861 Sidney Herbert, now seriously ill, went to the Lords and it was left to Lord de Grey to carry out the Herbert reforms. Miss Nightingale hoped that this would mean that the military hospital being built at Woolwich would be a true general hospital and would be lifted out of the petty jealousies of the regimental system.[9] The Herbert reforms were looking towards a comprehensive army health service, but this was something which the military minds could not encompass. As soon as Sidney Herbert was dead the Duke of Cambridge pressed for the cancellation of the Woolwich hospital but Lord de Grey stood his ground and, at Miss Nightingale's suggestion, it was called the Herbert. When the hospital was nearing completion Mrs Shaw Stewart was asked to be the superintendent with Colonel Wilbraham as the governor. At first she refused, seeing it as a move to get her away from true bedside nursing, and there followed much eccentric correspondence. It is not clear whether the post being offered was 'Superintendent General', but at last Mrs Shaw Stewart accepted and Miss Nightingale wrote:

> Mrs Shaw Stewart has accepted the Superintendence as I expected showing her inconsistency by a long letter of abuse of me to Lord Herbert, which really seem to have nothing to do with it and stipulating that the nurses should be C. of E. which he granted. Both she and he are legally wrong as the regulations give absolute power to the Superintendent in this respect – which she knows. Please say exactly what she said to you about returning all her letters to her, I am ready to do but I don't want her to take it as an insult.[10]

These are presumably the letters which Professor Smith says Miss Nightingale 'evaded a specific request to return'.[11] What Dr Sutherland advised is not known but it certainly appears as if Miss Nightingale wanted no animosity. It is not clear exactly when the Herbert was opened. There was an opening celebration on 1 November 1865 and in 1866 *The Times* reported that there were 300 patients in the Herbert and '19 out of 20 disliked female nurses being thrust upon them'.[12] However, it seems that Mrs Shaw Stewart and her team may have nursed in the Old Garrison Hospital at Woolwich where they had their quarters.

While awaiting the opening of the Herbert Mrs Shaw Stewart, with a group of nurses she had personally recruited, established a female nursing service at Netley, but not without trauma. In 1862 Captain Douglas Galton, who had married Miss Nightingale's cousin Marianna, became an assistant under secretary at the War Office, and Douglas soon became the intermediary between the warring Major General Wilbraham and the angry and tempestuous Mrs Shaw Stewart. He arranged for the Major General to see Miss Nightingale.[13] In spite of Miss Nightingale's irenic proposals relations worsened and eventually at the end of May 1868 an enquiry was set up by the War Office and held at Netley. The tribunal consisted of Dr Sutherland, Dr Beaston and General Hay and lasted from 29 May to 9 June with the account occupying some 16 closely printed pages.[14] Two things stand out. First, the whole proceeding has a very modern ring and reads like many a Health Service enquiry in the past 30 years. Second, the doctors, and even friends like Professor Longmore, saw the nurses as the doctors' chattels. Having resisted the concept of nurse training they now expressed annoyance if particular nurses were neither trained in their techniques nor able to help with their particular operation. What also emerges from the enquiry and the correspondence was that here was a social divide. The patrician Mrs Shaw Stewart did not mingle with the doctors socially and her attitude to her nurses was equally aristocratic – it was her privilege to cuff them if they deserved it. In spite of the evidence that showed that Mrs Shaw Stewart's temper was at times uncontrollable, there was no criticism of the nursing and the moral tone was good. As Miss Nightingale put it 'the cooking was good in spite of the cook'.[15] Notwithstanding the intervention of her brother and friends in high places Mrs Shaw Stewart was forced to resign.

Miss Nightingale wrote to Sir Harry Verney, 'there has been a bagarre at Netley with Mrs Shaw Stewart compelled to resign and the W.O. want me [sic] to choose and train a superintendent and nurses'.[16] This was an indication that Miss Nightingale saw herself as synonymous with the Fund, and that when one door closed she did not repine but picked up the pieces and started again. Her personal nominee was out; she would now influence military nursing through the Fund.

It was at this juncture that the Fund became actively concerned with military nursing, an involvement that was to be fraught with difficulty. Miss Nightingale, in spite of Mrs Shaw Stewart's epistolatory abuse, remained loyal to her friend and held that her nurses were good. At Netley there were nurses to be accommodated and, once Mrs Shaw Stewart's strong presence was removed, the various military administrators moved in with recommendations, particularly on behalf of nurses who had been dismissed. Miss Nightingale, not unaware of male motives, wrote: 'I do not think the Fund should take any nurses dismissed by Mrs Shaw Stewart for I have always found her characters correct.'[17] The War Office said they had names of nurses suitable for training by the Fund and the Major General sent names to Mrs Wardroper direct which caused displeasure at the War Office.[18] In the general confusion possible candidates withdrew and Mr Bonham Carter, while accepting the War Office's choice of a superintendent for training, took a firm line: 'It is undesirable that the Fund should take nurses from Netley… the Fund will supply the necessary staff.'[19]

The choice of the potential superintendent was Mrs Jane Deeble aged 40 years, the widow of an army surgeon who had died in Abyssinia, who had three children and an army pension of £140. She was seen by Mrs Wardroper and taken on for training where she was reported to be a 'lady of superior abilities'. At the end of the training year, the Fund, with advice from Mrs Wardroper, selected six nurses for Netley: they were Mrs Rebecca Strong, Jane Kennedy, Jessie Lenox – all sisters – Lucy Emm who had been displaced at Liverpool and needed a job, Lucy Wheldon and later Ann Clark.

Before the team could leave for what Miss Nightingale considered to be the miasma-ridden marshes of Southampton Water, the Fund had to tackle the problem of providing accommodation for nurses, for Netley had not been built for female staff, nor indeed for the Army Medical College which also moved there in 1863. The War Office had to be bullied into providing quarters that were comfortable, seen to be respectable and totally secure. Both Mrs Wardroper and Mr Whitfield paid visits, but Miss Nightingale thought that neither understood the different requirements of a military hospital and she complained that Mr Whitfield merely said 'sick men are the same anywhere'. In a long and amusing letter to Henry Bonham Carter Miss Nightingale sets out the difference and, incidentally, offers a clue as to why the Fund made so much fuss about nurses' quarters at St Thomas's hospital:

> Every night, of every year, every military hospital contains a certain number of non-commissioned officers who are more or less the worse for drink... people think that the discipline in military hospital will be strict; it is not, it is worse than in civil hospitals.

She then relates stories about porters hanging around the stairs at St Thomas's and making themselves objectionable to the probationers – a fact that Mrs Wardroper did not seem to know – and goes on to entertain her cousin with her reminiscences of Scutari when she had to sleep with the key of the nurses' quarters under her pillow and the practical consequences of what happened if the key went astray. The Fund must insist on security, because she knew from experience that the military would not take action against soldiers found trespassing.[20]

Mrs Deeble and her group were due to go to Netley in October 1869 but in September the War Office confessed that the alterations were not complete, suggested a temporary arrangement, and, adding insult to injury, complained that the adaptions were costing £500. Mr Bonham Carter, now cast in the role of Mr Standfast, wrote unequivocally 'no secure quarters, no nurses' and suggested that the War Office, having made the agreement, should be responsible for paying the nurses from October. This seems to have had the desired effect and the alterations were promised for October.

By the time the team were ready to depart most of the formal female nursing staff at Netley had left and Miss Nightingale wrote with satisfaction 'General Wilbraham finds out that not withstanding his inclination to be the matron, and his experience for the post, he does not fill it successfully.'[21]

Another favourable development was the publication of the Regulations for the Royal Victoria Hospital, Netley.[22] These were the regulations referred to by Miss Nightingale in her letter to Dr Sutherland and were more or less drafted by the Fund and contained the all important clause that the superintendent was responsible to the Secretary of State to whom she reported and, above all, she had the power to dismiss a sister though the reasons had to be notified to the Secretary of State. These regulations with their 54 clauses were important because they became the issue of contention when the Fund later tried to negotiate the position of the nurses at the Herbert hospital. Once again the nub of the argument lay in accountability. In the 1868 Netley Regulations the Nightingale principle triumphed.

Before Mrs Deeble left for Netley Mr Bonham Carter took up her cause with the War Office who now proposed to reduce her pension by £90 per year, which meant she was accepting the responsibility of superintendent for a mere £60 a year. When letters did no good Sir Harry Verney took the matter direct with Lord Northbrook and the decision was reversed, Mrs Deeble was grateful and at this stage the atmosphere between her and the Fund was cordial. Miss Nightingale did not see Mrs Deeble until she was about to leave for Netley which indicates that she did not interfere with the selection of candidates and she did not see them all as biographers suggest. Her impressions are worth recording in view of the subsequent cool relationship, and as an example of Miss Nightingale's somewhat protean character assessments:

> I had more interest in her than I felt possible – she has great qualities those which enable a woman to bivouac and struggle as wife and mother, but not those which make able to govern and fit into an organisation like Netley, she seems to have no idea beyond a regimental hospital. I foresee that we will have to do half her work for her is she is to remain as superintendent. And yet I liked her.[23]

But a week later, after she was installed, Mrs Deeble returned with her little daughter and Miss Nightingale wrote that she was

> greatly impressed by Mrs Deeble's improvement, she shows more apprehension than I gave her credit for, she has mastered that 1. the D.G. and the Horse Guards will do nothing for her, it lies with the War Office and 2. a Military General is totally unlike a Regimental Hospital.

Then comes the very human postscript: 'And that heavenly little girl!! (She ought to be made the Superintendent General.)'[24] However, it is not long before both Miss Nightingale and Mr Bonham Carter are showing exasperation about 'doing half the work' and Mrs Deeble is told she 'must be responsible for selecting and recommending her staff'.[25] This was in spite of glowing approbation from General Wilbraham, which, one suspects, annoyed Miss Nightingale more than his antagonism to Mrs Shaw Stewart.

One of Mrs Deeble's first acts was to ask the Fund for a night superintendent because, having got the message about regimental hospitals, she was trying to break the 'Comrade system' whereby very ill soldiers were allowed to have a 'comrade' to nurse them particularly at night. Also she expressed the view that if she was to find suitable staff she must train them herself. This brought down coals of fire on her head and provoked the Fund into setting out why military hospitals should not be training schools. On the whole the reasons were sound, particularly the inadequacy of experience, and they were the reasons given against Service hospitals being training schools by the General Nursing Council some 60 years later. Nevertheless, it is difficult to see what else Mrs Deeble could have done in the circumstances in 1868. In-service training at Netley was better than no training.

Mrs Deeble's fall from grace seems to have been occasioned by the turnover of staff which brought an almost unbelievably sharp rejoinder from Miss Nightingale and Henry Bonham Carter, unbelievable because a high turnover and sickness rate was a feature of St Thomas's hospital. It had been true of Liverpool and was soon to be true of Highgate, all of which were headed by superintendents of the highest moral tone. In January 1871 Mrs Deeble wrote to say that the work was becoming heavier, that Emm had been dismissed and she was looking for a replacement, and that sisters Clark, Kennedy and Strong had all been ill.[26] Since Miss Nightingale had predicted illness because of the poor site, the damp and the walking of long distances it is a little surprising that Mrs Deeble should have been censured. Then came the blow that sisters Kennedy and Strong wanted to leave and break their contract with the Fund. Mrs Strong wrote that she would forfeit her third year gratuity and her certificate.[27] In spite of Mrs Deeble's letters saying that she had talked to both sisters and pointed out their duty and tried to persuade them to stay, quite unusually Mr Bonham Carter drafted a censorious letter starting 'Dear madam' and going on:

> There will be a meeting of the Fund Council and it will be reported that you entered Netley with six carefully selected nurses; one nurse has been dismissed, two have given notice and you report another being discontented and the Committee will attribute this in some measure to the Superintendent... even allowing for the difficulties...[28]

It is to be hoped that the actual letter was kinder than the draft.

Mrs Deeble could not only bivouac, she could defend herself. It appears that Mrs Strong was unhappy because of her husband who had left her, and Mrs Strong wrote to say that Mrs Deeble had given her great support. Kennedy was angling for a better job and now, belatedly, Miss Nightingale admitted that Emm should never have been sent, that 'Strong was nervous' and 'they should have considered the husband's existence' and that Kennedy was always 'self seeking'. Nevertheless the damage was done and the relations between the Fund and Mrs Deeble were never good again. But by now Mrs Deeble had the approbation of the War Office and the Fund's displeasure need not have bothered her.

Mrs Deeble kept her three sisters and Emma Berry, sent by Mrs Wardroper, who herself confessed she had not enough education to cope with the doctors' demands, and she took staff from other hospitals and did her best to give them some training, later taking staff from other training schools. The Nightingale connection with Netley slowly came to an end. Miss Nightingale continued fearing that Mrs Deeble would make a fool of herself with the War Office and go the way of Mrs Shaw Stewart, and Miss Torrance was sent to advise. Miss Torrance was fond of Mrs Deeble but is alleged to have said that Mrs Deeble 'might think herself too powerful and write an indiscreet letter', however, we only have Miss Nightingale's version of what Miss Torrance said.[29]

In spite of these forebodings Mrs Deeble seems to have kept the support of the War Office, carved herself out an empire and in 1881 had an advertisement in *The Times* offering training to a limited number of nursing sisters who were under the aegis of the National Aid Society. During the Zulu War in 1882 she took 14 nurses to South Africa, eight to Pietermaritzburg and herself and the rest to Addington. Later, sisters from Netley served in the Egyptian campaigns including the Sudan war. In 1883 the War Office reorganised the service and gradually Netley trained nurses were found at the Herbert, the new Cambridge Hospital, Devonport and Malta. From time to time there are letters from Mrs Deeble to Miss Nightingale reporting progress, most of which only produced sarcastic comments. Mrs Deeble finally retired in 1889 and is generally regarded as having laid the foundations for the Queen Alexandra Royal Army Nursing Service.

Miss Nightingale's attitude to Netley and Mrs Deeble is difficult to understand. Of Mrs Shaw Stewart she has said 'if some of the things related had happened to me, F.N., I should have felt the same. Only my feeling would have been expressed by a laugh – hers by rage.'[30] Mrs Deeble was the opposite of Mrs Shaw Stewart; she managed to get on with the doctors, the irascible Major General and the War

Office and, instead of being delighted that peace reigned, Miss Nightingale was furious – did she think it betokened compromise? Could it be that no one should manage the War Office but FN? When the cold shouldering of Mrs Deeble is compared with the latitude and sometimes inordinate affection displayed to other Nightingales like Machin and Williams, one can only conclude that Miss Nightingale expected more from the military nursing than was reasonably possible with the resources of the time.

Once there was a rift in the relations between the Fund and Netley Miss Nightingale dropped the idea of a Superintendent General; 'until we have two superintendents there can be no Superintendent General', she wrote. There was, however, another more formidable reason why there were now no trained female nurses at the Herbert hospital. Although Lord de Grey had carried through some of the Herbert reforms the tripartite and internecine organisation of the War Office remained. In the interregnum between these and the more drastic reforms of Edward Cardwell in 1871, the Horse Guards, under the diehard Duke of Cambridge, reasserted themselves and the Herbert hospital lapsed into the pernicious old regimental system. Miss Nightingale wrote: 'The Herbert was intended as a General Hospital but it has become regimental. The change under considera-tion is to be made at Netley, the only one suitable for the training of nurses.'[31] This was a comment which indicates that by 1872 Miss Nightingale may have changed her mind about Mrs Deeble training nurses. Nothing, however, could be done about the Herbert for the simple reason the Fund was not invited to do anything. After the Shaw Stewart 'bagarre' the Fund was ignored. Sir Harry Verney was asked to speak to Mr Cardwell, who was by now Secretary of State for War, and to suggest that Mr Bonham Carter might come and discuss the Herbert situation with one of the under secretaries. Such a meeting presumably took place because by 1876 the dialogue started again.

In the meantime Mr Cardwell had done for the army what Sir Charles Trevelyan had done for the Civil Service. The buying and selling of commissions between regiments was abolished and above all there was a reorganisation of the tripartite structure of the War Office which was replaced by a tidy linear line of communication and chain of command. The cherished Netley regulations did not fit into this plan. Once again dispute and delay were about accountability. However, it seems to have been the War Office's intention to upgrade the Herbert as a General Hospital and introduce female trained nurses, but before the Fund would co-operate it had to fight the battle for the supremacy of the superintendent all over again.[32]

By June 1876 negotiations between the War Office and the Fund were far enough advanced for Mrs Wardroper to discuss furnishings for the proposed quarters with Mr Bonham Carter. Emmeline Stains was chosen as acting superintendent and two more sisters, Miss Shillington and Miss Enderby, went to the Herbert in September. At this point Henry Bonham Carter received an extraordinary letter from the War Office:

> The quarters for the superintendent and nurses are not yet completed. The moment everything is ready I will let you know and we will make a beginning. Sir Wm Muir will be much obliged if you will arrange for the removal of the nursing sisters with us now.[33]

This was a letter which taxed even Miss Nightingale's powers of sarcasm.

The unfortunate sisters were duly 'removed', not pleased that they were losing opportunities for applying for posts elsewhere. But it was not only the nurses' quarters that were at issue; when the final proof of the Herbert Regulations came they were totally unacceptable to the Fund. The winter – of considerable discontent – was spent hammering out a compromise. Eventually the War Office agreed to pay the nursing staff the same scale as at Netley, but it remained adamant that the superintendent must be subordinate to the Principal Medical Officer, and there the matter rested.[34] At last a conciliatory move was made with the War Office emphasising that although termed PMO this officer was not resident and there was no question of the nursing superintendent being responsible to a Resident Medical Officer for day-to-day nursing matters. Finally, Miss Nightingale agreed:

> We should be disposed to compromise viz: 1. in order to afford the superintendent access to the Secretary of State she should be instructed to transmit all communications through the P.M.O. – who is the government. 2. Orderlies be instructed to receive instructions from the nurses in all matters relating to the sick. 3. Complaints against orderlies to be made to the medical officer in charge.[35]

In January 1877 Mr Bonham Carter saw Sir William Muir, the Director General, and expressed dissatisfaction with the regulations, comparing them unfavourably with the regulations the Fund had helped to draft for Netley. However, Sir William pointed out that

> Since the rules for Netley were framed a new organisation for hospitals has been established by the Secretary of State under which nursing sisters cannot be exempted from the control of the medical officer.[36]

By March another compromise was found and Miss Stains was again invited to be superintendent and to take with her Misses Ashton,

Shillingford and Enderby, all well-educated women with good reports but all needing employment. When at the end of April the War Office was still not willing to receive them they protested. Miss Ashton wrote that after the delay she felt obliged 'to decline to have anything further to do with the Herbert'. Miss Stains was more forthright: she said that she was applying to Wolverhampton and that 'the whole affair can be nothing but a ridiculous failure'. Mrs Wardroper also expressed dissatisfaction.[37]

In vain did Mr Bonham Carter urge patience – the women were adamant. Miss Stains became the matron of Wolverhampton and later the superintendent of the district nurses in Liverpool; Miss Enderby and Ashton went to Liverpool Infirmary, and Shillingford went home. Mr Bonham Carter wrote to the War Office: 'The Committee regrets having to withdraw nominations and have no others to recommend.'[38] The War Office were, no doubt, not entirely sorry.

As far as the Fund was concerned it never succeeded in altering the nursing at the Herbert and little improvement was made until Miss Caulfield from Netley became superintendent and insisted on having nurses already trained in civilian hospitals and on having proper rules and regulations and a pension scheme. Miss Caulfield also insisted on the need for army nursing sisters to be 'Superior educated persons' that they might command the respect of the soldier.[39]

The Fund was now effectively shut out of the Herbert and Netley, but a spur to reformed nursing in the army came from another quarter. In 1861 Henri Dunant had founded the International Red Cross in Geneva, and in 1870 the Franco-Prussian War with its horrifying stories of hardship and suffering brought home to people the inadequacy of the official provision for the sick and the wounded. In England the National Society for Aid to the Wounded was founded and £250,000 raised by public subscription. The Society – subsequently the British Red Cross Society – sent aid to both sides and Miss Nightingale somewhat unwillingly became involved, unwilling because she said there 'were more lives to be saved in India' and, one suspects, because she thought that armies should have their own official welfare and nursing services. Because of her friendship with Victoria, the Crown Princess of Prussia, Miss Nightingale was first concerned with the German cause and sent Miss Florence Lees, who had been an observer at the Nightingale School, to join Clementia Rumff, who had also done a spell with the Fund, and who had been sent to England by the Crown Princess. In spite of having been earlier declared by Miss Nightingale as 'totally unfit for superintendence' Miss Lees apparently acquitted herself well.[40]

The National Aid Society under Lord Wantage (Colonel Robert

Lloyd Lindsay) had on its executive Sir Harry Verney, his daughter Emily and Sir Douglas Galton, while Henry Bonham Carter and Dr Sutherland were sent on a tour of the French and German hospitals. The Nightingale influence was not missing. However, sending supplies was one thing, but when the Society started to recruit and talk about 'trained' nurses that was another. With the outbreak of the Zulu War in January 1879 the National Aid Society asked for a superintendent and 12 nurses to be sent to the seat of war. Asked for advice Miss Nightingale was wary; to whom would these nurses be accountable? Where were they to be stationed? What would their relationship be to the nurses going out from Netley? Perhaps Miss Nightingale had memories of Mary Stanley's party descending on her at Scutari.

The following year the likelihood of war and the need for nurses increased at the other end of Africa. With its acquisition of shares in the Suez Canal Britain had a direct stake in the politics of Egypt and because Mr Gladstone, unlike his predecessor, was unwilling to call in the Turks, British troops had to be sent to crush the revolt by Arabi Pasha. Unfortunately the bombardment by the Navy led to a further uprising which later spread up the Nile.

The National Aid Society worked closely with the War Office – in fact Miss Nightingale suspected that 'Colonel Robert Lloyd Lindsay of the National Aid Society was trying to relieve Lloyd Lindsay of the War Office of spending public money on official nursing services.' The Society offered to pay for 'trained' nurses for Egypt, which threw into relief the vexed question of who was a trained nurse? The Director General obviously regarded the military nurses at Netley as 'trained nurses'. Miss Nightingale wrote in disgust:

> Does he call nurses 'trained' at Netley? Training there has been an utter failure and at the Herbert it has not been tried. Is Mrs Deeble to be the training superintendent of the women recommended by her at the Herbert?[41]

Mrs Deeble for her part, who after 12 years seems to have known how to look after herself, persuaded Sir Thomas Longmore of the Army Medical College that Netley was the only place capable of training army nurses, and she said that she knew from her own experience that at St Thomas's the dressers did the dressings. This was reported back to Miss Nightingale and it is a measure of her antagonism to Mrs Deeble that she entered into a long and unedifying correspondence with Mr McKellar of St Thomas's asking him to support the fact that the nurses at St Thomas's *did* many of the dressings. She wrote triumphantly to Sir Harry that Mr McKellar had supported her and had said that 'At Netley the majority of the patients were chronic sick and were up and about, if they had dressings they did them themselves.'[42]

This was all of little avail because the War Office persistently, and perversely, recognised Netley as the main recruiting base and training ground for army nurses. In 1882 Mrs Deeble was asked to take staff to Egypt. Miss Nightingale, annoyed, wrote to Mr Bonham Carter saying 'pray advise me what to do', a sure sign that she was tempted to do something intemperate. There is more than a hint of petulance in 'As far as I can see I have to take orders from Mrs Deeble.'[43]

Mr Bonham Carter and Sir Harry advised restraint. Mrs Deeble had the backing of the War Office and she particularly wanted to take Mrs Fellowes who had trained at the Nightingale School. Miss Nightingale made sure that it was not only Mrs Fellowes who was taken: Mrs Deeble must not be seen to dictate to her. In the end Mrs Deeble did not go herself but was replaced by Miss Helen Norman who has been trained at St Mary's by Rachel Williams, who was accompanied by Misses Solly, Airy, Winterton and Mrs Fellowes.[44] As it happened the campaign was short, with a victory at Tel-el-Kebir the war was over and in December Mrs Fellowes and Miss Solly rebelled and asked to come home, which they did while Sybil Airy stayed and continued to nurse in the military hospital in Cairo.

In 1883 the regulations for the Army Medical Department were rewritten and allowed for a superintendent of nurses with a staff of trained nurses to be appointed by the Secretary of State on the recommendation of the Director General to 'General and other hospitals'. The duties of the nurses were confined to the hospitals to which they were sent and 'they were to receive orders from the medical officer and all reports and communications were to be submitted through him to the Principal Medical Officer for consideration by the Director General'.

This was a negation of the compromise hammered out during the Herbert negotiations and Miss Nightingale's comments, running to many pages, were bitter,[45] as well they might be because the struggle had gone on for over 20 years and the position of nurses with regard to accountability seemed no better than when she had left Scutari.

In 1885 trained nurses were once again able to show their value to the army. In 1884 the War Office recalled General Gordon who was a friend of Miss Nightingale and to whom he had introduced his cousin Mrs Hawthorne, who had taken a great interest in military hospitals abroad, and was appalled at what she found – particularly in respect of the indisciplipine and neglect by the orderlies. Miss

Nightingale persuaded her to make a report and her account, with
other evidence thrown up by the war, was to form a basis for the
Commission of Enquiry of 1882.[46] In the meantime General Gordon
had taken charge of the garrison at Khartoum and held out against the
forces of the Mahdi, but because relief was delayed the garrison fell
and Gordon was murdered. This led to a bitter censure of the army
high command and it was against this background of criticism that the
Commission made its report.

In February Lady Rosebery, Mrs Gladstone and other ladies from
the National Aid Society called on Miss Nightingale and she agreed to
join the Princess of Wales's Branch. There were already female nurses
in Egypt from the last campaign and it was now proposed to send Miss
Rachel Williams, the 'Goddess', and a team of nurses. Interestingly
enough several years before Miss Nightingale had rejected Rachel
Williams as a candidate for the Herbert 'because she would fight with
every trained woman in the place and she has such a tongue with the
medical men'. Since Miss Williams's stay at St Mary's had been fairly
stormy (see Chapter 9) the early assessment may have been partly
correct. Before the campaign was over Miss Williams was writing to
The Times about the failure of army chaplains to conduct prayers on
the wards. Miss Williams took with her several Nightingale Fund
trained nurses, Philippa Hicks and Mrs Dowse (née Torrance) who
remained at Suez, and Miss Machin who had resigned from
St Bartholomew's and who with Miss Digby went to Souakim. Miss
Airy was already in Cairo.

Miss Nightingale took a great interest in the Fund's nurses who
went to Egypt and in the campaign itself. She went with Sir Harry
Verney to Victoria station to welcome his nephew's regiment back
from the first Egyptian campaign, and she was in her element organising uniforms, parting gifts, farewell breakfasts and comforts for the
journey, and of course, once the party had left there was the indefatigable letter writing. She wrote with every mail and there are 65 letters
to Rachel Williams alone which were in due course bequeathed to the
Fund.[47] But running through the correspondence there is a wistful
note – she would have liked to have been there herself. The letters not
only give advice on military nursing and the need for tolerance but
those to Rachel Williams contain a mine of gossip about the comings
and goings at St Thomas's hospital and of 'poor Mrs Wardroper's
tearful state' and the current intrigues at the War Office. The
Nightingale favourites were always part of the Nightingale family and
Rachel Williams was asked to contact Herman Bonham Carter who
was with his regiment at Souakim; this she apparently did and sent a
glowing account to her mother of 'how well he had done by his men'.

Like the first campaign the war was short and the party came home, though Sybil Airy was shipwrecked *en route* where she showed considerable courage and presence of mind.[48] Miss Williams came home engaged to Mr Daniel Norris and Miss Machin was soon to be married to Mr C. Redpath and go with him to South Africa. The original first Specials were now leaving the fold, Miss Nightingale began to feel old and her interest in 'her nurses' was never the same again.

The Commission of Enquiry eventually reported. Its findings were mild considering some of the horrifying evidence it had received; nevertheless it advocated that 'improvements in the system of nursing are both practical and desirable'. From now on nurses from Netley, supplemented by nurses from the various training schools that had sprung up around the country, were to be found in the five military hospitals in England and in Malta.

This situation was the background to the formation of the Queen Alexandra Imperial Nursing Corps after the Boer War. The death of the royal obstructionist, the Duke of Cambridge, and the Royal Commission of 1890 paved the way for further reforms in the Army Medical Department. When Mrs Deeble retired Miss Norman took over as the Lady Superintendent with 19 superintendents under her. There was a rapid increase in numbers and, under the patronage of Princess Christian, a reserve corps was built up and in 1898 the Army Medical Department was reorganised into the Royal Army Medical Corps. Princess Alexandra of Wales, who had always taken an interest in army nursing, had herself organised and despatched nurses from the London Hospital to the seat of war and had initiated the Red Cross Medal, among the first recipients being, ironically enough, Miss Nightingale and Mrs Jane Deeble. Finally, after the death of Queen Victoria, the army nursing service was reorganised as an amalgamation of the existing services based on Netley, and the Military Nursing Service for India, the scheme under the National Aid Society having come to an end.

To the end Miss Nightingale remained slightly hostile; she was critical of the army nursing service in a way that she was not towards other nursing ventures. She makes statements without supporting evidence: 'Military sisters, with exceptions, are much below the best hospital sisters and their superintendent, Miss Norman is by no means a first class woman.' By now Miss Nightingale was 74 years old and critical of nursing generally, but there is no reason to suppose that the nursing sisters who went to the Boer War were not highly regarded.

Miss Nightingale and the Fund were never successful in establishing a military nursing service on the lines laid down in the *Subsidiary Notes*. The main reason was that until after the Egyptian campaigns the War Office was not enthusiastic about having female nurses. As

Miss Nightingale said it was 'as if the Crimea had never been', a denial, if one were needed, of the steady progress-towards-the-light theory. Moreover, the War Office certainly had no intention of having women in the army not accountable through the normal channels. The Fund was adamant that in matters of nursing discipline the superintendent must be supreme, so they were bypassed. However, apart from matters of principle in the early years there was the sheer practicality of finding enough trained nurses of the right calibre, and it was not until nursing had become 'fashionable' that this could be done.

Nevertheless, no attempt at reform is entirely lost, and when eventually a military nursing service was established as a corps some 40 years later the principles were those laid down for military nursing by Miss Nightingale. The matron-in-chief was responsible to the War Office, all nursing staff were trained in civilian hospitals and only those of 'sister' calibre were recruited; for many years the age for recruitment was 28 years or more. Miss Nightingale's vision of what a military nursing service should be, as she planned it after the Crimean War, came true in the First World War.

Notes

1. Ridley, J., *Lord Palmerston* (Constable, London, 1970), p. 430.
2. *The Builder*, 'Netley Hospital', by Miss Nightingale, 4 July 1858; Cook, Sir E., *Florence Nightingale*, vol. 1, p. 431.
3. Ridley, *Lord Palmerston*, p. 518.
4. Nightingale F., *Subsidiary Notes as to the Introduction of Female Nursing into Military Hospitals in War and Peace* (Harrison & Sons, London, 1858).
5. Ibid.
6. J. Sutherland to FN, BL, Add Mss 45792, 14 January 1857, f. 14.
7. Woodham-Smith, C., *Florence Nightingale*, pp. 478 and 245.
8. J. Sutherland to FN, BL, Add Mss 45751, 6 January 1856, f. 168.
9. FN to J. Sutherland, BL Add Mss 45751, January 1861, f. 168.
10. FN to J. Sutherland, BL Add Mss 45792, July 1861, f. 195.
11. Smith, B.F., *Florence Nightingale – Reputation and Power* (Croom Helm, London, 1982), p. 155.
12. Piggot, J., *Queen Alexandra Royal Army Nursing Corps* (Leo Cooper, London, 1975).
13. FN to Capt. Galton, BL, Add Mss 45762, 4 February 1864, f. 27.
14. *Official Report of War Office Enquiry Held at Netley*, BL, Add Mss 45774, May/June 1868, ff. 101–17.
15. Woodham-Smith, *Florence Nightingale*, pp. 478-80.
16. FN to Sir H. Verney, *Claydon Papers*, ? June 1868.
17. FN to H. Bonham Carter, GLRO, HI/ST/NC18.14(9), 24 October 1868.
18. FN to H. Bonham Carter, ibid., 14(10), October 1868.

19. H. Bonham Carter to Sir E. Lugard, ibid., 14(13) (draft), November 1868.
20. FN to H. Bonham Carter, ibid., 14(15), 1 October 1869.
21. FN to H. Bonham Carter, ibid., 14(21), 10 June 1869.
22. Printed *Regulations for the Female Nursing Staff at the Royal Victoria Hospital, Netley.* GLRO, HI/ST/NC18.15(3a).
23. FN to H. Bonham Carter, GLRO, HI/NC18.15(51), 1 November 1869.
24. FN to H. Bonham Carter, ibid., 15(59), 7 November 1869.
25. FN to H. Bonham Carter, ibid., 15(11), 3 December 1869.
26. Mrs Deeble to H. Bonham Carter, ibid., 18(6), 22 March 1871. See also Summens: *Angels and Citizens* (Routledge, London, 1982).
27. R. Strong to H. Bonham Carter, ibid., 18(6), 22 March 1871.
28. H. Bonham Carter to Mrs Deeble (draft), GLRO, HI/ST/NC18. 18(9), 27 March 1871.
29. FN to H. Bonham Carter, HI/ST/NC18, 18, 21, 12 January 1871.
30. Woodham-Smith, *Florence Nightingale,* p. 479. See also Cook, *Florence Nightingale,* vol. 2, p. 66.
31. FN to H. Bonham Carter, GLRO, HI/ST/NC1/72/29, October 1872.
32. Webb, R.K., *Modern England* (George Allen, London, 1969), pp. 340–1.
33. Sir W. Muir to H. Bonham Carter, GLRO, HI/ST/NC18.23(12), 29 September 1876.
34. H. Bonham Carter to Sir W. Muir, ibid., 23. (17–20), October 1876.
35. Sir W. Muir to H. Bonham Carter, FN to J. Sutherland, ibid., 23. (1), 15 February 1877.
36. Sir W. Muir to H. Bonham Carter, ibid., 23. (3), 26 January 1877.
37. E. Stains to H. Bonham Carter, also Ashton, Enderby and Wardroper to H. Bonham Carter, ibid., 23. (20–28).
38. Henry Bonham Carter to Sir W. Muir, ibid., 23. (33).
39. Piggott, J., *Royal Army Nursing Corps.*
40. Cook, *Florence Nightingale,* vol. 2, p. 203.
41. FN to H. Bonham Carter, BL, Add Mss 47720, 16 August 1880, ff. 105–7.
42. FN to Sir H. Verney, ibid., 1 August 1882. f. 253.
43. FN to H. Bonham Carter, GLRO/HI/ST/NC18.F 253, 1 August 1882.
44. FN to H. Bonham Carter, GLRO, HI/ST/NC1./82, 12 & 13, 29 July 1882.
45. FN to H. Bonham Carter, BL, Add Mss 47720, December 1883, f. 249ff.
46. Cook, *Florence Nightingale,* vol. 2, p. 337.
47. Letters to Egypt contained in the collection. GLRO/HI/ST/NC3SU180, 1–186.
48. S. Airy to FN, BL, Add Mss 45775, 15 June 1887, f. 148.
49. FN to H. Bonham Carter, BL, Add Mss 47726, 2 May 1894, f. 9.

7. District Nursing

Never think that you have done anything effectual in nursing in London until you nurse not only the sick poor in workhouses but those at home.

Florence Nightingale, Private Notes, Easter Sunday, 1867

In answer to the challenge that the Fund had been devoted exclusively to hospital nursing and mainly to the benefit of St Thomas's, Miss Nightingale said our answer must be 'to train training staff in Hospitals where they can be trained in order that they may train in their turn nurses for the sick poor of every description'. However, she went on to confess that she thought the answer was difficult to justify.[1] In the same letter she wrote:

> my view you know is that the ultimate destination of all nursing is the nursing of the sick in their own homes... I look to the abolition of all hospitals and workhouse infirmaries. But it is no use to talk about the year 2,000.[2]

During 1866 there was considerable correspondence about district nursing schemes and when philanthropists in Norwich wrote to the Fund for advice about setting up a scheme Miss Nightingale referred them to the Liverpool experience.[3] Apart from the fact that she considered hospitals to be corrupting places and 'a hard necessity of an inferior civilization'[4] the specific need for nursing in the home had been brought home to her by her early correspondence with Mr Rathbone.

Mr Rathbone's first wife had died of consumption in 1859 and she had been well nursed by a Mrs Robinson from St Thomas's, a proof, if one were needed, that not all nursing before 1860 was bad. Mrs Robinson so impressed her employer that she was persuaded to stay on and nurse the sick poor in their homes in the surrounding district, but the need was so great that she was overwhelmed and Mr Rathbone, realising the futility of one nurse among so many, decided to consult Miss Nightingale about promoting a general scheme for 'district' nurses for Liverpool.[5]

Miss Nightingale gave the Liverpool scheme much thought.[6] Although she helped in formulating a plan whereby Mr Rathbone financed a Nurses' Home built near the Liverpool Hospital where nurses were to be trained for work in both the hospital and the district, she was later somewhat caustic about the results, mainly, of course, because in 1860 there was no one to train the nurses. However, the Liverpool experiment is important because its organisation, with its Ladies Voluntary Committees, set the pattern for other District Nursing Associations and was the reason for the schism in ideas about planning and training district nurses at the end of the century.

Mr Rathbone, his second wife and his circle of Nonconformist friends were steeped in the ideas of the Charity Organisation Society, and their emphasis was on welfare rather than trained nursing care. To further his experiment Mr Rathbone sent two ladies, the Misses Merryweather, to St Thomas's as observers, but apparently neither was interested in promoting nursing as a separate skill. Under the Merryweather superintendence nurses were 'trained' to work in the Liverpool Royal Infirmary and in the 18 districts into which Liverpool had been divided. The system was set out in a long letter from Mr Rathbone to Arthur Clough.[7] After explaining that they were waiting for Sir Joshua Jebb, the chairman of the Fund Council, to give advice on the Nurses' Home, Mr Rathbone stated that they had spent £13,000 on improvements and that the hospital now had 19 wards and 230 beds. They intended having one Lady Superintendent but with the wards divided into 'sets' with one senior nurse in charge of each group of wards who would be responsible for the teaching of the probationers under her. Miss Nightingale commented in the margin that this was a poor arrangement because the probationers would not be moved around for experience. Mr Rathbone goes on to what was to be the crux of the district organisation, that as they found nurses

> suitable for missionary work on the district we will offer them to ministers of religion and other efficient, kind people in different wards of the town who will form local committees and raise among themselves funds for medical comforts and find proper superintendence; £16-£40 paid by the institution (who would retain certain control over the nurses) and £100 raised by each committee would go far to relieve a great deal of the most pressing nursing [needs] from sickness in Liverpool.[8]

It is clear that in spite of the fact that in later years Mr Rathbone said, 'in any matter of nursing Miss Nightingale is my Pope and I believe in her infallibility', the scheme he produced flew in the face of Miss

Nightingale's first principle that nurses should be accountable to a trained nurse with the nursing superintendent accountable only to the employing authority. How the Liverpool scheme worked out in fact is shown by a letter from Charles Langton, secretary to the Liverpool District Nursing Association, a few years later. Mr Langton, having explained that the work was essentially with the poor and destitute who lived in courts and cellars with many families in one house, went on to say:

> In about half the districts we have trained nurses, others are worked by women partly trained, or by reason of long experience qualified for dealing with those for whom they labour. Under the superintendent [illeg.] ladies' committee there is a lady inspector who goes round and enquires for herself into the generally efficiency of the nurse. Some superintendents prefer all untrained nurses, others cannot afford the expense. It is desirable not to fetter the ladies who supply the funds, and who have enough to do to satisfy the demands made on them. Relief is often needed more than nursing care, though the border line is some-times difficult.[9]

Mr Langton was probably right in that the primary need was generally economic and the poor were sick because they were poor. But the letter epitomises the dichotomy in attitudes between the professional and the voluntary workers which was to characterise so much of the early district nursing work. The 'ladies' often preferred untrained nurses because they did not argue or make conflicting decisions about the patients, and the ladies had to have their way because they provided the funds. Those who raised the money decided how it should be spent.

Interestingly enough the correspondence with Mr Langton was promoted because Miss Nightingale was trying to persuade all cities to use a standard form for home nursing cases.[10] Mr Langton sent a specimen of the returns saying, with considerable prescience:

> unless the medical profession generally is sensible of, and admits in prac-tice the value of such a return, we must perforce, in some degree, fail in our object... the ladies dislike statistics and object to the nurses filling up these forms.[11]

This objection did not cease in 1869.

In 1874 Mr Rathbone, who was now a Member of Parliament, wrote to Miss Nightingale about starting a District Nursing Association in London and Miss Lees, who had returned from the Franco-Prussian War, was suggested as a superintendent. Although Miss Nightingale was most anxious to do something about district nursing the request brought forth a portentous six-page letter in which set out her objections. These included the fact they had not enough data to know whether such as Association was necessary and that she thought that Mr Rathbone misunderstood the functions of such an organisation, confusing it with a welfare society; in forthright language, she complained of the Liverpool system where she said 'the nurses did no dressings, no bed linen changing, but they simply gave and the cases [patients] liked it'.[12]

The upshot of this criticism was to employ Miss Lees to do a survey of the systems of nursing in the various London hospitals in 1874 and to look at the current nursing practices by the different sisterhoods, religious organisations and other associations. The survey was thorough and extensive and is covered by corrections and additions by Mr Bonham Carter, so it is assumed that he assisted. The result is somewhat tendentious but nevertheless it gives a useful picture of the nursing situation in London around 1874, and with the usual Nightingale precision there is a printed questionnaire.[13]

Needless to say the St Thomas's training system receives the most praise, but good marks were awarded to the Middlesex which was training probationers and had nurses from the British Nursing Association, to University College Hospital which had sisters from All Saints and to King's College Hospital and Charing Cross, both of which had sisters from St John's House. St Bartholomew's, Guy's and the London were said to have no training system and were all dismissed with derogatory remarks. The results of the survey eventually appeared as *The Report of the National Association for Providing Trained Nurses for the Sick Poor*,[14] a booklet of 119 pages. This report contains much factual information and although the statistics in the 12 appendices may be suspect they are valuable source material. The survey of the District Nursing Associations currently operating in London, of which 11 supplied trained nurses, showed that there were 26 District Nursing Institutions in London. These included the St John's sisterhood who were trained at King's College and Charing Cross Hospitals, the British Nursing Association who trained at the Middlesex and the Royal Free Hospitals, curiously enough the East London Nursing Society whose nurses did a year's training at the London Hospital, and the Bible Women's Mission and the Mildmay Park Institute, who trained their nurses at Guy's. The report is contradictory about the training facilities at both the London and Guy's Hospitals, although it is certainly true that Guy's did not claim to start a training school until after the appointment of Miss Burt in 1879.[15] The report offers little factual evidence as to the value of the different schemes; instead it launches into the preconceived notion that there was a need for a District Nurse Training scheme in London which would include 'some knowledge of anatomy and physiology, methods of arresting haemorrhage and elementary chemistry'.

In April 1876 Miss Nightingale wrote a letter to *The Times* asking for support for the Metropolitan and National Nursing Association for Providing Trained Nurses for the Sick Poor which had been founded the year before with the Duke of Westminster as its first chairman. The letter to *The Times* was reprinted as a pamphlet in which Miss Nightingale set out the objectives of the Association:

> to bring a truly national undertaking – real nursing, trained nursing to the bedsides of cases wanting real nursing among the London Sick Poor... [this would be done by] providing a real home within reach of their work for nurses to live in... a home where any mother would be willing to let her daughter, however attractive and highly educated, live.[16]

The Committee of that Association was impressive. Headed by William Rathbone it included Poor Law experts like Nassau Senior and Dr Sieveking and medical men of the calibre of Henry Acland; above all it included the tidy mind of Mr Bonham Carter whose hand can be seen in the precise way in which the first report was set out. On the aims of nursing education for district nurses it emphasised that 'even the Nightingale School had not produced a systemic training', and 'students should be received at stated intervals with planned medical instruction and periodic examinations'.[17]

The 'classing' system was something for which Mr Bonham Carter had asked at St Thomas's for 14 years without success. Mrs Wardroper and her successors were so pushed to use probationers as the labour force that 'classing' did not really occur until St Thomas's accepted the idea of a Preliminary Training School in 1910. However the passage on High Class Nursing seems to have come from Miss Lees who was the secretary: 'Even the improved training at St Thomas's does not supply the comprehensive education and training that would elevate nursing to the rank of a scientific art for educated women like the medical profession.' To support this the report goes on to quote Dr Harvard of Montreal who said that nurses required 'a liberal preliminary education at least equal to that required by a medical student'. Miss Nightingale's disapproval of such sentiments is expressed in a letter to Mr Bonham Carter:

> She [Miss Lees] wrote to me herself. She says that we should make the nursing profession attractive to ladies by giving a higher training because ladies more than common women – as she calls them, are attracted to St Thomas's. But I did not point out this little inconsistency – the object is to encourage her (the lady) to work.[18]

It seems likely that some of the subsequent difficulties between Miss Lees and Miss Nightingale centred on the difference of their aims for nurse training. Miss Lees's views were dangerously near those that were soon to be expressed by the British Nurses' Association and the 'Registrationists'. On the other hand, when she was criticising the Liverpool system, Miss Nightingale had said, 'Two things strike me with force. (1) we do nothing to *train to train* (2) after talking to Miss Merryweather they do nothing either to train or govern district nurses.'[19] Miss Nightingale herself was to write:

> The District Nurse must first nurse. She must be of a yet higher class and of a yet fuller training than a hospital nurse, because she has no hospital training appliances to hand at all... the doctor has no one but her to report to him. She is his staff of clinical clerks, dressers and nurses.[20]

The Report of the Association was acted upon and in 1875 a Central Home was set up in 23 Bloomsbury Square with Miss Lees as superintendent and soon there were subsidiary Homes in Holloway and Paddington. Arrangements were made with the Nightingale Fund to train 12 probationers as Specials for the Metropolitan and National Nursing Association and in 1877 the Fund contributed £167 6s 6d to the Association and nine Nightingale nurses became trainees in the Home. The following year the contribution was £240 and seven nurses went from the Fund to the Association.[21] This pattern continued until Miss Lees married in 1878, after which the link became weaker, but the Fund was largely instrumental in launching the Association and contributions continued until 1881, the Fund always advertising the Association in its official report. There is reason to believe that Mrs Wardroper never wholly approved of the scheme and at one stage she wrote emphatically 'St Thomas's does not train for District work', and she apparently did not like Miss Lees who during her brief stay at St Thomas's 'did not submit to the regulations'. In 1875 Miss Crossland, who had become the Home sister at St Thomas's, wrote to Miss Nightingale about the wisdom of going to tea with Miss Lees for fear 'dear matron might object'.[22]

One Nightingale nurse who went to the Home in Bloomsbury was Mary Cadbury. She had been given three months' notice by Mrs Wardroper although apparently the parting was mutual. Mary Cadbury was a Quaker who wrote home regularly to a large and affectionate family in Birmingham in the most vivid and down-to-earth manner, and, fortunately, 205 letters have been preserved.[23] Mary Cadbury went to Bloomsbury in 1878 and her letters bring home the extent of the suffering in the homes of the poor, especially, sadly, among the sick children who of course were seldom admitted to hospital for fear of infection. Although saddened Mary was resilient, or perhaps not wanting to alarm her tender-hearted mother too much, and she gives a blow-by-blow account of her wrestles with feather beds, drunken fathers and the devices for getting nourishment into a bronchitic old man, all interspersed with stories of the fog of London and the doom of the Sunday sermon. But to all intents and purposes Mary loved her work and she seems to have found the atmosphere freer than in the Home at St Thomas's, where one senses she had not always been happy in spite of forming strong and supporting friendships with the other Specials in her year.

Prior to her marriage with the Reverend Dacre Craven – a worker for Poor Law reform – relations between Miss Nightingale and Miss Lees had become strained. There were obviously factions within the committee and it appears that Mr Rathbone and Miss Lees wanted to recruit Lady Probationers only, and at one stage there was a clash between Mr Bonham Carter and Mr Rathbone. Miss Lees constantly appealed to Miss Nightingale and apparently used her name in vain in committee. In March Miss Nightingale wrote:

> My dear Harry,
>
> I do not know what to do with this letter [from Miss Lees] except to ask you. I see that we will have to set up a training school for district nurses ourselves – a very good way of spending part of our capital. But for the life of me I know no one who could start the district nurses on their duties but Miss Lees...[24]

Here was an indication that Miss Nightingale was becoming disillusioned with the internal dissension, but a few weeks later she was writing of Miss Lees:

> She is treating us scurvily and has been doing this for seven years, a mixture of flattering, want of common consideration and truth – most nauseous. But for all that she is the only person who can do the work... It is impossible to forward to her what men say of her most justly.[25]

Evidently Miss Nightingale did try to tell Miss Lees what 'men', presumably her committee, said about her, but although Miss Lees was shocked 'self devotion had gone too far that it had little effect'. The following year there were more disagreements within the committee, and now Miss Lees imagined Mr Wigram to be conspiring against her. As usual Mr Bonham Carter tried to pour oil on troubled waters but at last even his equanimity was disturbed and he exploded: 'O women! women! what a curse you are in matters of business.'[26]

However, there is no doubt but that Miss Lees was able, and from the content of her lectures it is clear that she herself was skilled in a number of techniques. Bearing in mind that she had only been an observer at St Thomas's for four months it indicates that it was possible for determined, educated ladies with private means to get tuition, as did Mrs Shaw Stewart, and from the technical point of view they could bid fair to rival the medical profession which was itself a point of controversy. Moreover, contumacious though she may have been, Miss Lees held firmly to the view that the district nurse must be a trained and educated woman responsible only to a trained nurse superintendent, and in this she was at odds with the Liverpool system; for this, if nothing else, she deserves her place in nursing history.

In 1878 Miss Lees suddenly married the Reverend Dacre Craven; she was then 37 years old and he a well-known worker on various philanthropic committees. In 1888 he was invited to become a member of the Nightingale Fund Council which he served faithfully until he was forced to resign on grounds of ill health in 1917. After her marriage Mrs Dacre Craven continued to work for the Association and her book *A Guide to District Nurses and Home Nursing*, duly proof-read by Miss Nightingale herself and published by Macmillan in 1889, was long considered to be the standard textbook; always being noted in the Fund's reports. In the controversy over Miss Lees, as with so many of the disputes over Nightingale nurses, we have only Miss Nightingale's side of the story, and Miss Nightingale was given to exaggeration. Miss Lees's career before in the Franco-Prussian War, her apparently successful marriage and subsequent career tend to belie the picture painted by Miss Nightingale. Once again the question had to be asked, did Miss Nightingale expect too much of her superintendents and was she intolerant of any deviation from her own ideas on nursing?

In spite of the difficulties at the Metropolitan and National Association Miss Nightingale and the Fund continued to be deeply interested in district nursing. In an address to the Association in 1878 Miss Nightingale wrote:

> District Nursing, so solitary, so without cheer and stimulus of a big corps of fellow workers in the bustle of a public hospital, but also without many of its cares and strains requires what it has with you, constant supervision and inspiration of a genius of nursing and a common home. May it spread with such a standard all over London and over the whole of the land.[27]

The idea of the Central Home was developed and seen as pivotal to the scheme, rather like the Nurses' Home associated with hospitals. In a paper on district nursing written in 1880, Miss Nightingale recommended that every district nurse should do a year in hospital then three months or more district training, and that every two years district nurses should return to hospital for a three-month refresher course, a recommendation which, needless to say, was never put into practice.[28] The whole enterprise was to be under the control of a Lady Superintendent at the Central Home who would have under her district superintendents who would control and supervise the nurses attached to a District Home with whom the supervisor should have a 'real and continuous official and unofficial relationship'. The supervisor was more important than in hospital because it was important that the nurse should not be deflected into other tasks like almsgiving. In a memorandum Miss Nightingale asks the question which seemed to obsess working on the district at the time:

> Are district nurses to be doctors in any sense of the word? Indeed are there any real directions given by the doctor to the district nurse for care and treatment except in rare cases where the doctor sends for the district nurse. Has the nurse to run after the doctor? Does he make it possible for her to meet him by appointment at the patient's bedside?[29]

The comment on the failure of doctors to use the district nurse is interesting because it was to be made time and again by nurses and was last heard nearly a hundred years later in the Hockey Report.[30] However, the lack of co-operation and communication between the district nurses and doctors had an added importance at the time because so often the poor could not afford a doctor and they saw the district nurse as a substitute. This led to the argument that the services of the district nurse might deflect the poor from thrift and from joining a provident association, and doctors in poor areas sometimes saw trained district nurses as a challenge. But Miss Nightingale saw district nursing as more than just giving treatment in the home:

> Besides nursing the patient, she shows them in their own homes how they can call in official sanitary help to make their one poor room healthy, how they can improvise appliances, how their home need not be broken up.[31]

The remainder of Mrs Dacre Craven's superintendence was not always happy: there were difficulties with the district supervisors and at one point it looked as if the Association would have mass resignations on its hands. A Miss Myers wrote from Holloway complaining that

> Miss Lees had made accusations and no enquiry had ever been held [and she was therefore] sending in her resignation and returning her gratuity, in so doing I am placing myself beyond the condemnation of the Nightingale Fund.[32]

Mr Bonham Carter, who was on the Council of the Association and also treasurer to the Paddington Home, did his best to calm the fraught situation with Mrs Dacre Craven declaring that her resignation had been forced. Eventually Mrs Dacre Craven did resign and was replaced by Miss Mansel in 1887 who stayed but a short time and was replaced by another, and later well known, Nightingale Nurse, Miss Amy Hughes, who remained superintendent until 1894 when she went to Bolton.

In 1887 the Queen Victoria Diamond Jubilee gave district nursing a new boost. After much diplomacy and counter-diplomacy by competing interests, £70,000 (the greater part of the Women's Jubilee Offering) was given for an extension of district nursing schemes, and the money provided for the foundation of the Queen Victoria Jubilee Institute for Nursing the poor in their own homes. A provisional committee was set up with the Duke of Westminster and Sir James Paget as trustees, with Mrs Dacre Craven as one of the moving spirits, and with a niece of Mr Rathbone, Rosalind Paget, later Dame Rosalind, who had trained as a nurse at the London hospital, as the first Inspector General. Queen Victoria took an interest in what she called 'my nurses' and in the design of the distinctive uniform and badge worn as a pendant, of which Miss Nightingale did not approve.

In spite of the fact that Miss Nightingale wrote a gracious intro-duction to William Rathbone's *History of District Nursing*, which was prepared for the Institute,[33] and that schemes under the Institute were designed on the lines laid down by the Metropolitan and National Nursing Association, which eventually affiliated with the Institute, and both Mr Rathbone and Mr Bonham Carter were closely involved; letters suggest that the relationship with Miss Nightingale was not always happy. It seems that she feared that district nursing was just becoming a job and 'the fashion', and that the need for a long training would be sacrificed to expediency. Professor Smith suggests that Henry Ponsonby and William Rathbone combined to stop Miss Nightingale getting hold of the Jubilee Fund in order to underwrite her plan for training district nurses. They wanted to use part of the money for a superannuation fund with which it is implied that Miss Nightingale disagreed. It seems possible that Miss Nightingale did want the money to be used for training, as indeed much of it was, but she was by no means against a superannuation scheme. She was always insistent on writing pension rights into contracts of service and she applauded Sir Henry Burdett's scheme which was always mentioned in Fund Council reports.[34]

By 1890 it is suggested that Miss Nightingale was getting somewhat arteriosclerotic and that she tended to be almost paranoid on some subjects, one of which was a 'Register'. Having fought a battle with the British Nurses' Association, and gained a tactical victory she seemed to see 'registers' where none existed. Just as she now found the nurses at St Thomas's 'Louder and nastier'[35] so she found the Queen's Institute as

> nothing but a register for quack nurses... there is insufficient inspection and that nurses straight from training are sent where they are needed by a Committee and not where they are needed from their training point of view.[36]

As a criticism of the Queen's Institute this is a little hard considering it was the complaint by Miss Nightingale herself for the past 30 years about the training school at St Thomas's. The same kind of jaundiced outlook comes out in her proof-reading of Miss Hughes's book where she crosses out 'profession' and puts in 'calling' and disputes the need to boil milk – this some 15 years after Koch had discovered the tubercle bacillus – and is scathing about antisepsis.[37] However, on another occasion, she is equally scathing about Miss Gordon, the Matron of St Thomas's, and Miss Crossland who had not accepted the need for antisepsis 'because they do not want to hear anything new'.[38] One can only conclude that at this stage (1896) Miss Nightingale's views were a little erratic.

In fact the Queen's Institute did foster a high standard and promoted professional nursing on the districts as opposed to the Associations outside the Institute who were often run and controlled by Ladies Welfare Committees. The Nightingale Fund can claim to have helped with the foundation on which the Queen's Institute was built and they continued to encourage their nurses to enter this form of nursing by advertising the Queen's Institute in their reports until the Second World War. Far from being a register for 'quack nurses' by the end of the century there were only 539 trained Queen's nurses, but they were the shoulder on which the great District Nursing Service of the twentieth century was to stand.[39]

Notes

1. FN to H. Bonham Carter BL, Add Mss 47714, 4 June 1867, f. 204.
2. FN to H. Bonham Carter, ibid., 4 June 1867, f. 203.
3. FN to H. Bonham Carter, ibid., September 1867, f. 258.
4. FN to Wm. Lavers, *Claydon Papers*, 20 January 1869.
5. Rathbone, W., *The Organisation of Nursing in a Large Town*, with an introduction by F. Nightingale (Longmans, Green & Co., London, 1865). See also Stocks, M., *A Hundred Years of District Nursing* (G. Allen & Unwin, London, 1960).

6. Cook, Sir E., *The Life of Florence Nightingale* (Macmillan, London, 1913), vol. 2, p. 125.
7. W. Rathbone to A. Clough, BL, Add Mss 45795, 6 June 1860, f. 13ff.
8. Ibid.
9. Chas. Langton to FN, GLRO, HI/ST/NCV69, 11 January 1869.
10. Printed instructions about the use of forms for home nursing. GLRO, HI/ST/NC15.
11. Chas. Langton to FN, GLRO, HI/ST/NCV/69, 11 January 1869.
12. FN to H. Bonham Carter, BL, Add Mss 47719, 15 June 1874, f. 42.
13. *Nursing in London Hospitals*, compiled by F. Lees with notes by H. Bonham Carter. GLRO, A/NFC/22, 2, 3 and 4.
14. GLRO, HI/ST/NC15 13b, June 1875 (printed booklet).
15. Cameron, H.C. *Mr Guy's Hospital* (Longmans, Green & Co., London, 1954), p. 203.
16. *The Times*, Good Friday, 14 April 1876, p. 6, col. c. See also *Metropolitan & National Nursing Association for Providing Trained Nurses for the Sick Poor* (Cull & Sons, London, 1876), p. 11; also in *Selected Writings of Florence Nightingale*, compiled by L. Seymer (Macmillan, New York, 1954).
17. GLRO, I/ST/NC15 13b.
18. FN to H. Bonham Carter, GLRO, HI/ST/NC1, 74.4, 17 July 1874.
19. FN to H. Bonham Carter, BL, Add Mss 47719, 8 July 1877, f. 62.
20. Nightingale, F., *On Trained Nursing for the Sick Poor* (Cull & Son, London, 1876).
21. *Nightingale Fund Council Annual Reports 1876, 1877 & 1878.*
22. M. Crossland to FN, BL, Add Mss 47738, 15 September 1875, f. 7.
23. GLRO, HI/ST/NTS/Y/16.1. The Cadbury Letters.
24. FN to H. Bonham Carter, BL, Add Mss 47719, 1 March 1875, f. 71.
25. FN to H. Bonham Carter, ibid., 29 March 1875, f. 87.
26. H. Bonham Carter to FN, ibid., 1 January 1878, f. 138.
27. Miss Nightingale's address to the Metropolitan & National Nursing Association (GLRO/HI/ST/NC15, 13c), quoted in Tooley, S., *The Life of Florence Nightingale* (Cassell & Co., London, 1910), p. 203.
28. Nightingale, F., *On Trained Nursing for the Sick Poor* (Spottiswoode, London, 1881).
29. Ibid.
30. Hockey, L., *Feeling the Pulse* (Queen's Institute of District Nursing, London, 1966).
31. Nightingale, F., Introduction to the 'History of Nursing in the Homes of the Poor' in *History of District Nursing* by Wm. Rathbone, dedicated to Her Majesty Queen Victoria (Macmillan & Co., London, 1890).
32. Myers to H. Bonham Carter, BL, Add Mss 47719, 11 January 1878, f. 226.
33. Cook, *Florence Nightingale*, vol. 2, p. 356.
34. Smith, F.B., *Florence Nightingale – Reputation and Power*, p. 168. See also footnote in Cook, *Florence Nightingale*, vol. 2, p. 356.
35. FN to M. Crossland, BL, Add Mss 47741, November 1896, f. 267.

36. FN to H. Bonham Carter, BL, Add Mss 47726, May 1895, f. 158.
37. FN to H. Bonham Carter, BL, Add Mss 45813, March 1895, f. 124.
38. FN to a Finnish nurse, BL, Add Mss 45727, 23 May 1886, f. 84.
39. Baly, M.E. (ed.), *A New Approach to District Nursing* (Heinemann Medical Books, London, 1981), p. 282.

8. The Nightingale Nurses Abroad

> Your Bengal Sanitary Commission is doing work like men – like martyrs
> in fact, and what work it is! All we have in Europe is child's play to it.
> Health is the product of civilisation, i.e. real civilisation. In Europe we
> have a kind of civilisation to proceed upon.

Florence Nightingale to Sir John Lawrence, 1864

In the past nursing historians have been at pains to stress the missionary nature of the Fund's nurses and how the Nightingale system was
successfully exported to Germany, Sweden, India, Canada and
Australia. However the evidence does not support Lavinia Dock's
assertion that 'the early Nightingale nurses were especially selected by
Miss Nightingale for work in the colonies... they were a remarkable
group as is emphasised by every recollection of them'.[1]

One nurse was sent from Germany and one from Sweden to
observe at St Thomas's but neither in fact took back the system nor
started a school on the Nightingale pattern. In her work on India Miss
Nightingale put forward plans for a system of nursing with head
nurses trained in England and then sent to Madras and Calcutta,[2] but
the plan came to nothing and few Nightingale nurses worked in India.
Lucy Leighton went out as a missionary and died on the voyage out[3]
and later Miss Ashton went to Ceylon, but in 1865 such a scheme was
too costly. Even if the finance could have been found and the Fund
had the nurses, in India nursing was not a top priority and Miss
Nightingale knew it.

It was to the countries within the context of 'the kind of civilisation we
have in Europe' that the Nightingale message was predominantly taken,
namely Canada and Australia. This was partly because in the second half
of the nineteenth century emigration had an attraction for the more
adventurous spirits among women, and partly because of the demo-
graphic reason – there being half a million excess females in 1861 –

but largely because the Empire offered more social mobility and job opportunity. When overtures were made from the Empire the Fund Council welcomed the opportunity of gaining publicity and prestige. Miss Nightingale, urging Henry Bonham Carter to push at the War Office door, wrote:

> I believe if we could get more government engagements like Sydney – as India and the War Office would be, we could attract a higher class of woman that we can get to serve under piddling committees like the work-house of Liverpool.[4]

The army in Australia had contributed to the Nightingale Fund as had private individuals, so when Sir Henry Parkes, the Colonial Secretary to New South Wales, wrote to the Fund in 1866 about nursing in the infirmary in Sydney, Miss Nightingale felt impelled to accept on two counts, namely, gratitude and publicity.[5] There was of course a strong case for refusing because at that stage the Fund had neither a superintendent nor a team of suitable nurses available. At this point a Miss Lucy Osburn applied to the Nightingale Fund. Miss Osburn, aged 29, was herself distantly related to Miss Nightingale through one of those many cousins and had nursed in Vienna, Kaiserwerth, Holland and Jerusalem and was, as Mrs Wardroper put it, 'mistress of several languages'. There was one difficulty: Miss Osburn's lawyer was her cousin, John Carr, and he objected, as others had done, to the Fund's contract. He wrote to Henry Bonham Carter, who was of course also related, saying that it was 'a most objectionable thing such as no lady ought to be subjected to... '[6] After considerable doubt that Miss Osburn would arrive, a compromise was worked out and Miss Osburn did a shortened training with the view of going to Sydney as the superintendent. However, Miss Osburn's 'training' did include observation visits to Liverpool and to workhouse infirmaries which were presumably made at her own expense.

The arrangements for the Sydney team were made between the Nightingale Fund and Captain Mayne, the colonial agent in London, and it was agreed that the Lady Superintendent should be paid a salary of £150 and the sisters £50 with board and lodging and the return fare paid to London provided the three-year contract was fulfilled.[7] Again Mr Carr entered an objection, this time to the clause in the contract that 'increments should be payable on good behaviour'. 'Are such expressions introduced into contracts for gentlemen?', he asked with some justification. Unfortunately the reply is not preserved but presumably Miss Osburn's contract was modified.

After some delay Miss Osburn and five head nurses left England in December 1867. The nurses chosen by Mrs Wardroper were Mary

Barker, Helen Turriff, Betty Chaunt, Elizabeth Blundell and Annie Miller. Miss Nightingale herself took great pains to see that they were properly equipped for the journey and that they had a nucleus of text-books.

The Fund had been careful to spell out Miss Osburn's terms of reference; she was to have entire responsibility for women engaged as probationers, male nurses were to be discontinued, and although the Lady Superintendent was to be responsible to the medical officer for the treatment of the patients, she was directly responsible to the gover-nors for the cleanliness, ventilation, warming of the wards and the administration of diets and medicines, and for the delegation of those duties. The Sydney hospital had been in existence since 1830 but the previous matrons had been subordinate to both the doctors and the lay administrators, and, Miss Osburn, like others, had to carve herself an empire. Needless to say there were difficulties. The doctors interfered with the nursing and there was considerable conflict with the lay administrator. In order to avoid confusion over letters Miss Osburn tried to get her title changed to Lady Superior and the head nurses to 'sisters' but as Miss Osburn had High Church leanings the whole thing was interpreted as a Romish plot.

As Judith Godden points out, the Evangelicals were a powerful faction and dominated Sydney's charities including the Sydney Infirmary, and when the Lady Superior ordered the burning of some of the bug-infested Bibles there were accusations in the *Protestant Standard* and an official inquiry.[8] There were other problems: the promised new hospital was not ready, the nurses' sleeping quarters were bug and lice infested and, according to the Nightingale party, the hospital nurses and servants were dirty, slovenly and 'unprincipled and untrustworthy' while they themselves felt isolated.[9]

In March 1868, a week after their arrival, an assassination attempt was made by the Fenians on Prince Alfred, Duke of Edinburgh, as he paid an official visit to Sydney. The wounded Prince was nursed in the Sydney hospital by two of the Nightingale nurses, Haldane Turriff and Annie Miller, and Queen Victoria sent her thanks to the English nurses for the care of her son. This proved a splendid public relations coinci-dence for the Nightingale Fund as the Queen was about to lay the foundation stone of the new St Thomas's hospital.[10] Unfortunately Miss Osburn sent an indiscreet letter about the wounded Prince to her cousin, Mr Carr, who circulated it in London clubs. The news fell on the horrified Fund Committee like a bombshell and Miss Osburn offered to resign.[11] As it happened the letter was suppressed and Miss Osburn withdrew her resignation but the harm was done. Hereafter

Florence Nightingale referred to Lucy Osburn in the most disparaging manner, coupling her with others who fell from grace like Miss Kidd, Mrs Deeble and Miss Barclay, as examples of women who had been placed in Superintendent's posts without adequate training, and all of whom had been rushed into positions because the Fund needed the publicity.

Miss Osburn soon earned further displeasure because she continually reported to Mrs Wardroper and Miss Nightingale, as she was urged to do, on the failings of the nurses she had brought with her, all of whom had had favourable comments in the Red Register.[12]

> You ask me for a report of the sisters I brought with me: pray don't Mr Carter, for I could not give it. I daresay they would make excellent nurses but it puts them in a false position to make them Sisters, and they have not borne the strain. So many of the nurses [local] are better educated... the only chance the sisters have of keeping their position is by quiet dignity, in this too often they have failed and my personal influence is daily exerted to prevent the nurses from openly showing contempt... Mary Baker is the best... Bessie Chaunt having secured her lover is quiet enough now – these two do not ride rough shod over the nurses nor enrage the doctors... of the other three I had better say nothing for little good can be said.[13]

Lucy Osburn complained frequently of the sisters' flirtations with patients, wardsmen and doctors: 'Bessie Chaunt was the talk of the hospital and if she were not married she ought to be.'[14] She did marry; the baby was born three months later. Annie Miller was accused by Turriff, who was also writing complaints to Mrs Wardroper, that she was having 'a courtship with a House Physician who was a married man'. However, as Dr Godden points out, our main source of this information is Mrs Wardroper and that Miss Nightingale had thought that 'one of Mrs W's faults was a mania [for] seeing flirtation and marriage in everybody'.[15] On the other hand it is possible that Osburn and Turriff were overstressing the faults in others and the difficulties they faced in order to emphasise their own success.

At the end of the three-year contract all the sisters were dismissed by order of the Colonial Secretary, Henry Parkes, and only Lucy Osburn and Mary Baker were re-employed. This was a blow to the Nightingale Fund which Lucy Osburn compounded by inferring that the nurses she recruited in Australia were preferable to those sent out from England by Mrs Wardroper. Strangely enough there is not a word about Miss Osburn's scandal, or of the dismissals of the nurses, to be found in Mrs Wardroper's reports and the Sydney enterprise was conveniently forgotten. Cook, presumably prompted by Bonham Carter, accounts for the dispersal of the Nightingale team in Sydney by saying:

> Their services were too much appreciated. In a few years time all five had either married or received valuable appointments elsewhere and Miss Osburn had to recruit her staff from the Colony itself. Miss Nightingale thought that the expedition had 'failed'.[16]

The truth is that the one nurse praised by Lucy Osburn, Mary Barber, returned to Edinburgh in 1876 and found favour with Miss Pringle. Blundell and Chaunt married, which appears to have been their main object in life, but Turriff and Miller, trading on the approval of Prince Alfred and the shock the assassination attempt had caused in Australia, did find appointments elsewhere. Miller went to Brisbane but resigned in two months because of disagreements with doctors and then joined Turriff at Melbourne, who on the strength of being a Nightingale had obtained the post of matron at the new Prince Alfred hospital. Miller, it appears, quickly faded into obscurity. Haldane Turriff on the other hand lasted ten years at Melbourne but her career was marked by disputes with the doctors and charges including the accusation that she had 'an ungenial and repellent demeanour towards other officials'. She did not start a training school and left in 1880 to marry the auditor.[17] No doubt she had many provocations but viewed as a group the 'Sydney enterprise' do not seem to have been suitable ambassadors for British nursing, and on the whole they were a quarrelsome and cantankerous lot.

Lucy Osburn herself, though vilified by Florence Nightingale, was soon to be lauded by Australian nurses as their founder. Watson in his history of the Sydney Hospital takes the view that the nurses from England were misled about the conditions and that they were only to be allowed on the female wards, Miss Osburn herself being the victim of sectarian spite.

Fortunately we have another side to the story supplied by Mrs Arthur Onslow, a cousin of Sibella Bonham Carter, who lived near Sydney and wrote to her cousin saying that Miss Osburn was a 'quaint, queer little woman much wrapt up in her sisters and we like her'.[18]

This however did not mollify either Miss Nightingale or Henry Bonham Carter whose worst fears were confirmed when a Mr Roberts, a surgeon from Sydney came to London and dined with the Bonham Carters. In a letter to Miss Nightingale Henry wrote:

> I stated to him quite openly how we stand with Miss Osburn and what opinion we had formed about her. He entirely corroborates. I regret to say that her utter failure in some respects is worse than I expected but at the same time he does not attribute to her quite the self-seeking motives which seemed to us apparent.[19]

It is clear that Miss Nightingale and Henry Bonham Carter had pinned on Miss Osburn that favourite appellation for Nightingale ladies who fell from grace, that of 'self-seeking'. But Mrs Onslow knew Mr Roberts who she described as 'a rather faddy surgeon who had left in sad trouble' and that:

> He and Miss Osburn did not pull well together. Two doctors the other day spoke in the highest terms and begged [Arthur] to help in defending her from the ill natured attacks of the evangelical party because she is supposed to be High Church. All who know her like her and people come out of hospital and say how comfortably they have been nursed... Harry should hear both sides.[20]

In assessing Lucy Osburn's contribution to nursing, recent research in Australia shows that an analysis of her register of nurses at the Sydney Hospital (1868–78) suggests that her claim to success was founded on a myth. The attrition rate was a little better than at St Thomas's but dismissals for misconduct were much the same (15 per cent Cf 13.6 per cent). However, in looking at the attrition rate, the cards were stacked against the matrons of the day. Nineteenth-century nursing was hard, the hours long, the discipline severe and hospitals themselves rife with infection, therefore the sickness rate was inevitably high. Nevertheless, it was important to preach 'success', and in Australia, as in England, publicity paid dividends.

Dr Godden suggests that the stereotype of the 'angelic Nightingale nurse' was enthusiastically adopted in Australia and a myth has grown up around Lucy Osburn similar to that about Florence Nightingale: 'The Osburn legacy to Australian nursing is highly problematical and deserves exploring not whitewashing.'[21]

Lucy Osburn returned to England in 1884 where she died at the age of 56 years from diabetes, from which she had presumably suffered for some time. In condemning her and the enterprise as 'an utter failure' Miss Nightingale tended to overlook the fact that she had been sent out with a team quite unfitted for the task ahead. Although she herself was soon to admit that Mrs Wardroper's reports were 'not worth the paper they were written on', she never seems to have felt any remorse that the Fund sent out a team so apparently inadequate for the task.

The Fund Council's second experiment in sending a team abroad arose from a request from Montreal. In 1874 the Committee of Management of the Montreal General Hospital resolved 'that it is expedient that a system of trained hospital nurses such as approved of in England, should be introduced into the hospital'.[22] In November the

Committee raised the subject again, this time in connection with the need to enlarge the hospital:

> the training of nurses by the institution would be of great public benefit and it would give the hospital an additional claim on the community. The Committee have entered into correspondence with a lady in England, and have good hopes of being able to make satisfactory arrangements if the governors give sanction to the undertaking.[23]

The lady was Maria Machin, 'the most spiritual of the Nightingales', though MacDermont suggests that it was Florence Nightingale who was first approached.[24] However, there is no evidence for this, and the first letter in the Bonham Carter collection on the subject is from Miss Machin to Mr Bonham Carter enclosing a letter from Charles Alexander, the Vice President of the Montreal Hospital, to Henry Bonham Carter which says:

> Dear Sir,
>
> You are doubtless fully aware that we have made a definite arrangement with Miss Machin to return to Canada to manage for us the Nursing Department of the Montreal Hospital. It is her desire and ours that she should have the assistance of four nurses... I ask you to allow four such as are under your care to come.[25]

Miss Machin's own covering letter makes it clear that the arrangements were well advanced and she would be going to Canada in the summer because she says that it is reasonable to suppose that if she is interested in the improvements the Committee should have her on the spot, and she goes on to say that she hopes to see Miss Nightingale that afternoon and that she will see Mr Bonham Carter at his leisure and discuss plans with him.[26]

It seems likely that Miss Machin, who was born in Sherbrook near Montreal and brought up in Quebec, was known to the hospital authorities and had kept up her Canadian connections. The other reason for supposing that the approach had been made direct to Miss Machin is a letter from Miss Nightingale to Henry Bonham Carter enclosing 'an unsatisfactory letter Miss Machin has received from Montreal' but Miss Nightingale complains, 'she cannot be prevented from leaving and she proposes to go in the summer'. It is unlikely that Miss Nightingale would have selected Miss Machin, for her loss as Home sister to the Nightingale Home would be irreparable, for she had not long been installed and was regarded as the one person who could keep the peace with Mrs Wardroper.[27] Mr Bonham Carter, with legal caution, advised Miss Machin not to bind herself and to get her passage money assured. But what both Miss Nightingale and Mr Bonham Carter were most interested in were the plans for the new

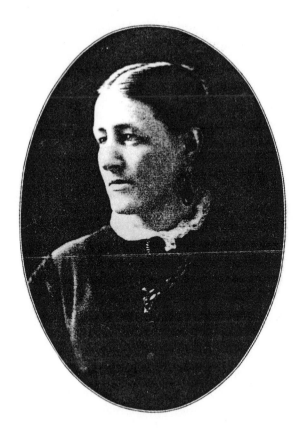

Miss Maria Machin in 1875

hospital and there is a vast amount of correspondence carried on through the agency of a William Whitford of Elm Court, Temple, who appears to have been the London agent for the governors. It seems that Captain Galton was consulted and considerable advice was given at the London end on the choosing of the site and the actual plans. It would also seem that the Fund, having had this project thrust upon them, hoped, as with St Thomas's, that they would be starting a School in a model hospital.

In May 1876 Miss Machin sent her belated report to the Fund Council. The reason for her delay was what she described as her 'anxious days', which was surely a euphemism for what must have been a terrible winter. Of her four nurses, Martha Rice had died of typhoid, Emma Randall had deteriorated and had neglected poor Martha when she was ill and had taken herself off and got married, Maria Sealey had too little education to cope, but Helen Blower was a valuable assistant and a good ward sister. Of the two replacements from England, Ann Marsh had typhoid and Jane Masters was failing to conform to discipline and was threatening to leave.[28]

Later, Miss Machin writes to say that there is a movement in the
hospital to start a training school for nurses and, although it is a far
from model hospital in which to start, she feels it would be a pity to let
the opportunity pass and has written to Miss Nightingale suggesting
improvements. In June 1877 she is writing to tell Mrs Wardroper that
she has gained permission from the Committee to send for two nurses
and that 'Mr Redpath would pay the passage out', and she goes on to
say that she wants nurses 'of a better stamp than Masters and
March.'[29]

Back in England Miss Nightingale apparently gave much thought
to the suggested improvements and came out against piecemeal
measures: 'No improvements or alterations could make the present
building into a good hospital, it is hopelessly unhealthy and it would
be throwing good money after bad to attempt it. Miss Nightingale's
advice was that the governors should acquire a new site and erect a
new 400-bedded hospital as quickly as they could with possibly T. H.
Wyatt as an architect and with advice from Captain Galton.[30]
However, in Canada the governors were complaining about the cost of
running the hospital in its present form and it is doubtful if they were
ever serious about rebuilding.

In spite of everything Miss Machin wrote home that she was happy
and receiving every kindness, she was stimulated to persevere and her
nurses felt the same. Then in September 1877, according to
MacDermont, Miss Machin's life was shattered because her fiancé,
'the brilliant young member of staff, died tragically from diphtheria'.
As Miss Machin was a serious and very religious woman aged 33 years
it is hardly likely that she entered into an engagement with an
unknown doctor shortly after her arrival back in Canada unless she
had known him before. One possible explanation for her determina-
tion to return to Canada, in spite of the unsatisfactory conditions of
service, is that she already knew Jack Cline. At all events Jack Cline's
death does at least furnish some explanation of the misunderstandings
of the next few months and perhaps why Miss Machin was willing to
return to England when she did.

At the time of Cline's death Miss Machin was being censured for
the excessive use of staff and for raising the running costs of the hospital. The report of the Committee agreed that the English nurses had
been a great service, but what was needed was 'a matron who would
check the extravagance and waste among servants' and, more sinis-
terly,

> the undersigned must now refer to the Lady Superintendent... whose
> term of engagement is about expiring. One of the main objects contem-
> plated when Miss Machin joined the hospital was the establishment of a

training school for nurses. This it has been impossible to put into force. It would appear, therefore, undesirable to make any renewed engagement with Miss Machin.[31]

Miss Machin was called before the Committee and evidently failed to satisfy them. But now the medical staff took up cudgels on behalf of Miss Machin and the English nurses. The Medical Board pointed out that the number of nursing staff was by no means excessive for what was needed for proper care, and that in the treatment of disease good nursing care was of the utmost importance. At the same time they strongly deprecated any action that would have the effect of substituting a non-trained matron for a skilled Lady Superintendent. The dispute between the lay administrators and the Medical Board was now out in the open and was taken up by the Montreal newspapers. Miss Machin herself wrote a very dignified letter dissociating herself from all such partisan discussion, and the Committee, in the face of such odds, decided to retain the services of Miss Machin who had now been joined by Jane Styring and Laura Wilson from England.

Miss Machin may have dissociated herself from the newspaper attacks on the unhygienic condition of the hospital, but in April she wrote a terrible saga to Miss Nightingale about conditions. There had been a leak in the furnace room and no one understood the pipes because they were so old. With greasy water flowing everywhere, they then found a cesspool in front of the kitchen door, and had it not been for an old drainpipe accidentally left in the proximity the whole basement would have been flooded with contaminated water.[32] Miss Machin, like her chief, may not have believed in the germ theory of infection, but she believed in hygiene and she had reason to be disturbed: four of her nurses had typhoid and one had died. Well might Miss Nightingale write 'it is the first duty of a hospital to do the patient no harm'[33] to which she might had added 'and the staff'.

The renewal of the contract was a Pyrrhic victory, the divisions were too deep to heal and in May 1878 the report announced the resignation of the remaining English nurses. To the last Miss Nightingale urged restraint, suggesting to Miss Blower that perhaps they were making too much of internal hospital intrigues: 'I have lived through many intrigues in the last 25 years and I am living through them still. Intrigues are not peculiar to Canada.'[34]

Although Miss Machin had considerable cause for complaint, inasmuch as she came expecting a new hospital to be started that year and that she would be given the opportunity to start a training school, the faults were apparently not all on one side. According to MacDermont the account books show that the turnover of staff was inordinately high.[35] Of course, like Agnes Jones, Miss Machin may have been throwing out rotten apples, but ruthless redundancies are hardly likely to win friends and there is reason to believe there was 'a lack of adaptability on the part of Miss Machin whose uncompromising purpose was to apply Nightingale principles of nursing care, at whatever cost and without much thought for diplomacy.'[36] Of the staff she brought from England she dismissed at least three and Maria Sealy is said to have led a rebellion and stirred up a faction bent on undermining Miss Machin's authority. Maria Sealey may have been a very unworthy character, but there is no doubt that there was disloyalty and intrigue with which Miss Machin did not manage to deal.

This unhappy story might be regarded as consequent on the unique conditions in Montreal were it not for the fact that to some extent the story is repeated in Miss Machin's three years at St Bartholomew's. In spite of going there by arrangement with the Fund and the governors, and much good will, her relationship with the governors was not particularly happy; although she lengthened the 'training' she failed to start a training school – this being left to a London trained nurse, Miss Ethel Manson, later Mrs Bedford Fenwick. There was a contretemps over her own and her deputy, Miss Vincent's, resignation, and in view of Miss Vincent's subsequent career one is inclined to give her version of the affair more credence.

It is said that Miss Machin returned to Canada when she left St Bartholomew's in 1881 but she obviously returned to England again because she went with Rachel Williams to Egypt in 1885. Later she married a Mr Redpath, with whom she went to South Africa, established a hospital at Bloemfontein, and subsequently nursed at Kimberly during the siege in the Boer War. She continued to write to Miss Nightingale and in 1889 there is a record that she joined the British Nurses' Association because she thought it would be useful 'with the private nursing home she was setting up'.

The Fund Council never claimed that the Sydney and Montreal ventures were successes. This is probably why (although there is a mass of correspondence) there is little hard evidence in this country about either scheme. Cook only gives Montreal a passing reference and Bonham Carter clearly thought the veil should be drawn over the whole episode. Nursing historians, on the other hand, have claimed that Nightingale missioners took reformed nursing to both Canada and Australia and have made much out of little evidence. Both schemes are interesting, however, because they demonstrate clearly the two main difficulties facing the Fund in its pioneering enterprises. First, was to find a superintendent who had the right leadership qualities and who was also a well-trained nurse. Neither Miss Osburn nor Miss Machin had much real training at St Thomas's. Miss Machin had a poisoned hand and was in fact on the wards for only three months. Both were chosen because of their ladylike qualities and their moral earnestness, both were very religious, but these qualities, as the Fund found with Agnes Jones, do not necessarily foster a bent for diplomacy. Both Miss Machin and Miss Osburn had to carve out a nursing empire and they tried to do it on English and Nightingale lines, probably too quickly and without sufficient regard for local susceptibilities although Miss Machin, of course, started with the advantage of being a Canadian. The other difficulty facing the Fund, at least in the first 20 years, was that there was little selection of probationers and Mrs Wardroper's reports were not reliable; many of the ordinary probationers from working-class backgrounds were simply not capable of standing up to situations where initiative and finesse were required. These nurses may have passed muster duly supervised at St Thomas's, but sending them abroad or into military service was a different matter, and in many cases they were a burden to the superintendent.

The lesson was learnt and hereafter the Fund did not attempt to send 'teams' abroad, nor is there evidence that they were invited to do so. By the end of the century there was no longer the necessity because there were other organisations like the Indian Nursing Service and the Colonial Nursing Service which could perform the function better.

Notes

1. Dock, L. and Nutting, A., *A History of Nursing* (Putnam's Sons, New York, 1907), p. 173.
2. Cook, Sir E., *The Life of Florence Nightingale* (Macmillan, London, 1913), vol. 2, p. 55.
3. GLRO, HI/ST/NTS/C4.2 (Number 39 in Book B).
4. FN to H. Bonham Carter, GLRO, HI/ST/NC18/15.4, December 1899.
5. Watson, F.J., *The History of the Sydney Hospital 1811–1911* (Gullick, Sydney, 1911).
6. J. Carr to H. Bonham Carter, GLRO, HI/ST/NC18/8, June 1866.
7. Watson, F.J., *Sydney Hospital.*
8. Godden J. England V. Australia – Lucy Osburn and the founding of Nightingale nursing in Australia 1868-84. Paper presented at Nursing & Women's History & the Politics of Welfare, Nottingham University, 1996.
9. Ibid, quoting Turriff/F. Nightingale, 1868.
10. Longford E., *Victoria R I* (Pan, London, 1964).
11. Watson, F. J. ibid. p. 451.
12. Maggs, C.M. (ed.) *Nursing History. The State of the Art. Analysis of the Register of Nightingale Nurses* (Croom Helm, London, 1985), pp. 47–59.
13. Osburn/Bonham Carter, GLRO HI/ST/NC18/10, 7 August 1869.
14. Godden, J., ibid.

15. Nightingale, F./Bonham Carter, H. July 1873 (quoted in Godden, ibid.).
16. Cook, Sir E., ibid., vol. 2, p. 192.
17. Paterson H *5 30am Nurse – The Story of Alfred Nurses 1871–1996* Victoria, Australia, History Books Chapter 1.
18. Onslow, Mrs/Bonham Carter, S. BL, Add Mss 47714.
19. Bonham Carter, H. /FN GLRO HI/ST/NCV 50, 72, 2 October 1872.
20. Onslow, Mrs A./Bonham Carter, S. BL, Add Mss 47717, 14 August 1872 f. 152.
21. Godden, J., *Stereotypes & Silences, Australia's First Nightingale Nurses* (Australian Society of the History of Medicine, Brisbane, 1996).
22. MacDermont, H.E., *The History of the School of Nursing of the Montreal General Hospital* (the Alumnae Association, Montreal, 1940), p. 17.
23. Ibid., p. 17.
24. Ibid., footnote.
25. Chas. Alexander to H. Bonham Carter, GLRO, HI/ST/NC18/12.26, 18 March 1875.
26. M. Machin to H. Bonham Carter, GLRO, HI/ST/NC18/12.27, 4 April 1875.
27. FN to H. Bonham Carter, BL, Add Mss 47719, 4 February 1875, f. 212.
28. Mrs Wardroper to H. Bonham Carter, GLRO, HI/ST/NC18/13.33, 4 September 1875.
29. M. Machin to Mrs Wardroper, GLRO, HI/ST/NC18/13.34, 22 June 1877.
30. FN to H. Bonham Carter, BL, Add Mss 47719, May 1875, f. 107.
31. MacDermott, *School of Nursing* p. 20.
32. M. Machin to H. Bonham Carter, BL, Add Mss 47719, 20 April 1877, f. 196.
33. Nightingale, F., *Notes on Hospitals* (Longmans, Green & Co., London, 1863), p. 1.
34. FN to H. Blower, GLRO, HI/ST/NC1/77, 11 October 1877.
35. Desjardins, S., *A History of the Nursing Profession in Quebec* (Association of Nurses of the province of Quebec, 1971).
36. M. Redpath to FN, GLRO, HI/ST/NC1. V6/89, 12 March 1889.

9. The Nightingale School Moves to Lambeth

The Fund has been devoted exclusively to the benefit of hospitals and almost exclusively to the benefit of St Thomas's.

Florence Nightingale, 1872

On 21 June 1871 the new St Thomas's was formally opened by her Majesty Queen Victoria and patients were admitted in September. Sir James Clark, who had been active in persuading Queen Victoria to perform the function, wrote sadly that if only the Prince Consort had lived the hospital would have been built in a more healthy situation.[1] However, it is doubtful whether Albert himself, with all his capacity for marshalling facts, could have persuaded the medical facility to move from the prestige of the centre of London; moreover, John Simon had astutely arranged for the Lambeth site to be bought on favourable terms.[2]

On the opening of the new hospital the Fund Council reported:

To provide an efficient nursing staff for so much larger a number of patients than have been accommodated at the Surrey Gardens was a work of considerable difficulty. The object being of essential importance to the well being of the training school, this Committee lent their willing endeavours to attain it. With this in view 18 probationers were placed on the hospital staff and four nurses were transferred to it from other situations. Of the above eight were appointed to be hospital sisters.

The Fund Council's records show that in 1870 there were only 18 probationers left out of the previous intake of 31, so this stretched resources and left no margin for other hospitals or schemes. Contrary to intention the Fund was indeed staffing St Thomas's. Of the eight who were appointed as sisters only three were with the Fund three years later. It so happened that the need was not so great as forecast. The Lambeth borough assessed the rates due on the new building as

147

£17,580 and although they were reduced to £12,500 the Court of Governors appealed to the Queen's Bench who ruled the hospital rateable at £8,100, but with five years owing. At the same time the governors faced a claim for dilapidations at Surrey Gardens and in order to meet costs wards had to be closed.[4] To make matters worse the running costs of the new hospital were proving to be the most expensive in Europe.

While the School was in the Surrey Gardens Miss Nightingale herself had little contact with it, her vast correspondence for that period is mainly directed elsewhere, and she did not see the probationers unless they were going on a special mission with which she was concerned. However, we do know from Mrs Strong that all the probationers were seen by members of the Fund Council, probably mainly Mr Bonham Carter and later Sir Harry Verney; we know from other sources that Mr and Mrs Bracebridge visited as did Sir Joshua Jebb and Richard Monckton Milnes, and both Sir John Clarke and Mr William Bowman were familiar with the Surrey Gardens layout. However during the first decade the Fund's main concern was to get a better agreement with St Thomas's, to ensure that the new hospital provided a proper Nurses' Home with suitable safeguards, and to get good publicity for the experiment so that they had a wider choice of candidates.

The Council and Miss Nightingale were aware that all was not well. There had been criticism that the Fund was financing the hospital, rather than nurse training, in both the *Pall Mall Gazette* and *The Lancet*.[5] Moreover there had been criticism from some of the probationers; Mrs Deeble had complained about the lack of teaching and had quarrelled with Mrs Wardroper about her demand that probationers should stand to attention when she entered the ward.[6] But as Miss Nightingale was soon to dislike Mrs Deeble she put down her criticism to a 'self seeking attitude'. Similarly a complaint from Mrs Rappe, a Swedish lady, who wrote: 'we did not learn from this or that at St Thomas's and there was not held a single lecture in anatomy or physiology whilst I was there', and who went on to say, 'I would not recommend anyone to go to St Thomas's'[7], was put down to the fact that Miss Rappe and Mrs Wardroper were antagonistic to one another. Other complaints were attributed to the inability of the probationers to put up with the necessary discipline and Mrs Wardroper was praised for weeding out the malcontents.

After 1867, partly because the pressure of other work was slackening and partly because she had found a more robust way of coping with her ill health, Miss Nightingale began to take a greater interest in the Nightingale School. Elizabeth Torrance, one of the first Special

Probationers, was appointed matron of the Highgate Infirmary in 1869 and in the course of taking up her assignment paid a number of visits to Miss Nightingale who liked her wit and ladylike manner. It seems that Miss Torrance was frank about the lack of teaching at St Thomas's because Miss Nightingale quotes her in retrospect saying:

> You put ill-educated women under the same circumstances of training as educated women, and you give them the temptation of boasting of sacrifice – which they don't make, and no opportunity is supplied them of knowing or correcting their ignorance or want of education, not even their bad spelling or writing, much less their want of higher things – religious knowledge and principle.[8]

According to Miss Nightingale she went on to say that there was a universal complaint about the sisters at St Thomas's who never gave instruction, and Miss Torrance agreed with Mrs Shaw Stewart that 'the main trainer and principle instructor at St Thomas's is a drinking woman'. At the same Miss Torrance warned that the Record books were misleading and 'entries were made with as much caprice as if a cat had made them'.

The sequence of events between 1869 and 1870 is not clear. Miss Nightingale must have discussed her fears with Henry Bonham Carter who, it seems, was already unhappy about Mr Whitfield to whom the Fund was paying £100 a year to give instruction. There had been the episode in 1863 when Mr Whitfield had been before the Court of Governors for misappropriation of supplies and at that time Miss Nightingale and Mrs Wardroper had rallied to his defence. However, Mr Bonham Carter was not naive and it was increasingly clear that the section at the bottom of the register, requiring the comment of the medical instructor on each probationer, was missing or subsumed in a general anodyne comment by Mrs Wardroper, who had said on a previous occasion 'we think as one'. It seems likely that it was Miss Torrance who first alerted Mr Bonham Carter to the more serious gossip about Mr Whitfield and the general opinion of Mrs Wardroper and the relationship between the two which apparently vacillated between staunch friendship and 'incessant quarrelling'.[9]

In July 1871 Mr Bonham Carter wrote that he had spoken to Mrs Wardroper about the register and he himself agreed with Miss Torrance's information:

> I am afraid the only good sister is Pringle. Should we make her Wardroper's assistant? [but] then she would be lost to the ward... It is useless to go on discussing Wardroper's defects except with a view to supplying the remedy... she cannot adapt herself.[10]

By the end of 1871, no doubt due to the publicity brought about by the new St Thomas's, there were a large number of enquiries from other institutions either asking for nurses or for advice on nurse training. It was now clear to Mr Bonham Carter that Mrs Wardroper was not capable of dealing with such correspondence, and more and more he himself took over:

> I don't think Mrs Wardroper is able to form a sound judgement [about nurses ready for superintendent's posts]. I have not thought it prudent to discuss questions which require a good deal of calm consideration.

He then proceeds to recommend both Miss Hill and Miss Barclay for senior posts.[11] In the same letter it is clear that Mr Bonham Carter was having serious thoughts about moving the school when the agreement ran out, or at least putting the Fund's eggs into different baskets for he continues:

> I would like to get hold of Poplar or Edinburgh Royal and perhaps something may be made of Belfast. Of the London hospitals the Middlesex would be most desirable. My endeavours to get a footing there some years ago failed and I did not get any response... Something might be done at the Royal Free and I should be glad to go over the Westminster.

The failure to get any response from the Middlesex relates to 1866 when the governors discussed starting a training school. After considering all the options they 'did not recommend that the supervision of nurses should be entrusted to anyone who was not chosen by the Governors and responsible to them'.[12] This was clearly an indication that not all hospitals wanted what might appear to be a cuckoo in the nest.

Early in 1872 Mr Bonham Carter saw Mr Whitfield with a view to getting his resignation from the School. In his defence Mr Whitfield said that for some time there had been a 'lack of cordial working together on Mrs Wardroper's side' and this he attributed to 'over excitement and irritability arising from the work and the changes of the last year and it was known to the sisters that his duties and hours had not been considered when arranging meetings for business'. In spite of his disappointment with Mrs Wardroper he was still willing to give assistance. On this reassurance Mr Bonham Carter presumably did not press the resignation issue, and he was unable to see Mrs Wardroper because she was ill in bed.[13]

In March 1872 it was agreed that Miss Torrance should leave Highgate and return to St Thomas's as Mrs Wardroper's assistant, that she should be replaced by Annie Hill, and that Miss Barclay, a well-educated Quaker, should go to Edinburgh as the Lady

Superintendent. Mrs Wardroper resented these proposals and Miss Nightingale herself interviewed the main actors in the drama (including Miss Barclay); from the information gleaned she wrote the long and revealing letter of 18 May 1872. Since much that happened later related to its content and to similar, and even more outspoken, letters extensive quotation is called for:

> ... But we are just in time to prevent Mrs W. from degenerating into a ~~hospital-scold~~ [Florence Nightingale's deletion] into governing like a virago. By talk, by being heard not felt. By speaking more than she observes all of which are almost the first elements of authority. She maintains authority by self assertion and she is losing it every day.
>
> What are we to make of this? She told me that she had told Mr W. that she was sure that his neglect had come to our common knowledge. I was forced to say; No – for if it had been he would not be there. I told her some things about his intoxication, she admitted it, but she did not choose to admit, or did not know all that I did. She said, almost without intending, that it was quite true that Mr W. had done nothing while Miss Rappe was there... To my unspeakable regret Mrs. W. told me herself that she had spoken to a probationer who had told her that Miss Cameron had ordered her out of the ward and said 'I can dismiss Miss Cameron and every woman in this place without referring to anyone'.
>
> This is true, but what a way to enforce authority. Miss Torrance may save her, but no one else can!

The letter continues with Mrs Wardroper's reasons for refusing to have Miss Torrance. First, Mr Whitfield objected: 'he almost said that Miss T should not come'. Then she put her own objections: if Miss Torrance was Mistress of the Probationers and came on to the wards to give tuition, that would undermine discipline, and she should be forbidden entry to the hospital.[14] This long letter from Miss Nightingale and others in a similar vein are important because they posed the great dilemma now facing the Nightingale Fund, which had a contract with St Thomas's and an undertaking to pay the matron and the Resident Medical Officer as instructors to the School; they had no power to dismiss them if they proved incapable, and they had no assurance that they would be consulted over new appointments – all they could do was to withdraw the Fund's support at the end of the contract. If they did that where would they go?

In her attempts to keep the peace and not offend Mrs Wardroper too much Miss Nightingale came up with a compromise – the idea of 'Home Sister' as a title for the assistant, which was by no means descriptive of the job she proposed, which was 'Mistress of the Probationers', or in latter-day parlance, director of nursing education and training. Mrs Wardroper was reassured that she was the matron of St Thomas's and also head of nurse training paid for by the Fund. This Janus attitude by Miss Nightingale put the 'Mistress of the Probationers' in an impossible position and it is small wonder that St Thomas's had four Home sisters in three years ending with Miss Crossland, an older woman who relied heavily on Miss Nightingale to keep the peace with Mrs Wardroper.

Peace at any price delayed the introduction of nurse tutors for 30 years or more. Interestingly enough, the emerging nursing profession embraced the idea of a Home sister, as a warden of the Home, with role and function that was a travesty of what Miss Nightingale intended.

The reason for this wretched state of affairs was attributed to the fact that Mrs Wardroper did not know the probationers: 'We have a matron who never addresses a word to them. She never comes into the Home unless there is a row.'[15] The other reason was that Mrs Wardroper had promoted old friends like Annette Martin, the Sister 'Extra' who ruled the Home, or favourites of the flirtatious Mr Whitfield like Sister Butler who had been involved in a scandal over patients' property and who was a mischief-maker. Of Sister 'Extra' Miss Nightingale said: 'Black ingratitude and evil speaking behind backs is the greatest sin, of this it is said that Mrs W. is unconscious.'[16]

However, the second part of this long letter is devoted to Mr Whitfield, for whom the greatest execration was reserved and who was seen to be the evil influence on Mrs Wardroper:

> Mr Whitfield has been for years in habits of intoxication. For years he has been in the habit of making his rounds at night (at a later hour that anything could justify having kept Sister and the Dispenser up until they could wait no longer) oftener tipsy than sober. This appears to be known to everyone in the hospital for years... At the same time his flirtations with Sister Butler were a current joke as she was absolutely unfit to be a sister and was only kept on by Mr W. For the past 4 or 5 years Mr W. has done nothing for the probationers except to exploit his position to the verge (and beyond) of impropriety. I am now convinced that 'nothing' is literally accurate. He has not even attended them when they were sick.[17]

The problem of Mr Whitfield resolved itself. Quarters had been found in the Nurses' Home for Miss Torrance and in the course of the negotiations Mr Whitfield wrote what Parsons describes as 'an impertinent letter' to Miss Nightingale:

> If I remember rightly in extolling the sitting room for the person who is to have the superintendence of the Home I have omitted to say that the walls are papered with highly arsenical green.

Practical Dr Sutherland wrote a note, 'tell him to varnish the walls'. But this was the last straw. Miss Nightingale cut Mr Whitfield out of her will and on 26 November Mr Bonham Carter interviewed Mr Whitfield and asked for his resignation. Mr Whitfield was told that his offer of resignation had better be renewed:

> I stated quite plainly that we had not had the assistance from him of late years which was due. He talked about resigning a year ago and I declined but the agreement we came to on the instruction he was to give was never acted on...[19]

But Mr Whitfield fought back and wrote to Miss Nightingale:

> I simply wish to ask what does the Secretary of the Nightingale Committee, what can he, seated in his office, know of the working details of the hospital. Worse than nothing... I had hoped Miss Nightingale would be spared the trial of witnessing the failure of plans which I clearly see must sooner or later follow their adoption, as I predicted the result on the abrogation of the apprenticeship.[20]

Well might Miss Nightingale write in the margin 'What can this man mean?'

However, to give Mr Whitfield his due, as a farewell gift he made a generous donation to the School of a mechanical skeleton, diagrams and books.[21] He left St Thomas's shortly afterwards and died in 1877.

In spite of the fact that Mr Whitfield's original support of the Nightingale Fund was not unconnected with personal ambition, in the early years he did attempt to give probationers some instruction, and he may have served the Fund well, but he seems to have grown disenchanted with the attempt. It was he who pushed Mrs Wardroper and for a time they worked in harness but, as the demands of the Fund grew greater and the School was visited by 'great folk', there were periods of mutual recrimination and at one stage, when Mr Whitfield's resignation was being asked for, Mrs Wardroper feared that Mr Whitfield 'would injure her because he was so vindictive'.

Mr Whitfield departed from any responsibility to the Fund but all was not well. Mrs Wardroper became more excitable and given to talking without purpose. Miss Nightingale wrote: 'If you could see her as I see her, because I can't take up my hat I am sure you might think her brain might go any day.'[22] Now, to make matters worse, Miss Torrance announced her intention of marrying Dr Dowse, the Medical Superintendent at Highgate. What Miss Nightingale said Miss Torrance said about wanting to get out of the engagement and what Miss Torrance actually said are probably two different things. Miss Nightingale was furious that Elizabeth Torrance, the linchpin of her plan, should desert, and Miss Nightingale declared that she was only marrying 'the wretched little Dowse to do him good'.[23] It could be that Miss Torrance, at the age of 35 years, preferred to be the wife of the 'wretched Dowse' to the impossible position that was being offered of responsibility without authority yet with confused accountability.

Miss Torrance took up her post in November 1872 and stayed long enough to reveal the muddle in the bookkeeping. Apparently Mrs Wardroper did not keep separate accounts for the Home and it seems possible that the Fund was subsidising the housekeeping for the ordinary nurses working at St Thomas's. Miss Torrance was of the opinion that 'the probationers were terribly hard worked and that the ordinary nurses had too little work' and if only Mrs Wardroper had been capable of laying out the work and making the nurses do their share then probationers would have had afternoon classes.[24] Another revelation was that the nurses left their patients and stood to attention before Mrs Wardroper when she was in the ward. Although Mrs Deeble had complained earlier, Miss Nightingale now believed her and was shocked.

In January 1873 Miss Torrance was taken ill and left before her six months had expired. There seems to have been some dispute about her final salary, but there is no doubt she was under great strain and was hardly allowed to see the probationers. She married Dr Dowse and, as was the case with a number of Nightingale favourites, she was subsequently disowned. Presumably Dr Dowse died because later Mrs Dowse wrote to say that she wanted to keep the Home in Hornsey Lane 'for the children' and use it as a nursing home; later she seems to have resumed amicable relations with Miss Nightingale and she joined the expedition to Egypt. There is nothing to suggest that Miss Torrance was not a reliable witness; she writes a good, educated letter and in general her story was corroborated by people like Miss Williams, Miss Cadbury and Miss Pringle, with whom she remained friends.

The relationship between Miss Nightingale and Mrs Wardroper at this stage is difficult to assess. There is evidence that once Mr Whitfield had gone Mrs Wardroper genuinely wanted to make a new beginning, she was remarkably loyal to Miss Nightingale, and Miss Nightingale always insisted that in spite of everything Mrs Wardroper had 'great qualities'. In the torrent of criticism that flowed between Miss Nightingale and Henry Bonham Carter for several years we have only Miss Nightingale's side of the story, though it does seem to be supported, rather less colourfully, by Mr Bonham Carter. But Mrs Wardroper must have been in an impossible position; she was matron of St Thomas's and responsible to the governors, and especially the treasurer, for running the nursing service for the whole hospital. Within that service she had 30–40 probationers who were employed by the Fund but who she selected and could dismiss and on whom she was now reporting to Miss Nightingale, some of whom were now 'lady probationers' and highly critical. To complicate matters the probationers, especially the Specials, were visiting Miss Nightingale and seeing Mr Bonham Carter, obviously discussing the faults they found in their training; this included the attitude of Mrs Wardroper and her inefficiency as a superintendent. Thirty-five South Street must have been a hotbed of gossip. Nevertheless there is no baulking the issue that at this stage stories of Mrs Wardroper's lack of interest in the probationers and her excitability and irrational behaviour abound. One possible explanation is that as she got older it was all too much for her; Miss Nightingale thought she was ill and wrote, 'Is the excitement a direct consequence of general ill health? but I doubt if any power will get her away.'[25] A hint that Miss Nightingale thought that Mrs Wardroper had changed comes in a letter to Henry Bonham Carter in which she says that Miss Barclay could not believe that 'Mrs Wardroper was ever different or that she ever had a serious notion in her head.'

Whatever the reason for Mrs Wardroper's apparent inability to cope, and whether Miss Nightingale was expecting too much and exaggerating the difficulties, it is important because the measures the Fund took to deal with the situation were to have consequences for the development of the nursing profession. Instead of taking the radical solution of removing the School and starting again they met the difficulty by a series of pragmatic measures. The most important was the installation of a Home sister who would take the care and tuition of the probationers out of Mrs Wardroper's hands. For reasons outlined the measure was only partial successful largely because the Home sister was not allowed into the hospital to teach on the wards. The concept was handed on that the head of nursing service must also be the head of nurse training – although she played no part in the training programme. A dichotomy that was exacerbated when the funding of nursing service and nurse education came from the same source – scarce hospital funds. With the advent of more doctors' lectures and a separate Sister Tutor the Home sister became more a warden and overseer of physical and moral welfare, but the post continued in the nursing hierarchy until the coming of the National Health Service when it was questioned whether this was not a waste of a nursing qualification.

The second suggestion that Miss Nightingale should move to Bird Cage Walk so that she could see the probationers more regularly was stoutly resisted by Mrs Wardroper, and not without reason. Mr Bonham Carter wrote that Mrs Wardroper had said that 'it would be subversive of her authority and the feeling would grow up that Miss Nightingale was to be looked upon as a superior officer'.[25] Mr Bonham Carter, who thought that there should be more involvement from Miss Nightingale, bowed to Mrs Wardroper's protestations and wisely condemned the plan of the house in Bird Cage Walk as unsuitable. Nevertheless it was agreed that the Fund Council should play a greater part in the affairs of the School and Miss Nightingale herself should see more of the nurses, although Mrs Wardroper was far from happy with this. Another innovation was that Miss Nightingale should write addresses to the probationers which should be read at a suitable occasion by a member of the Fund Council. Last, and by no means least, was the request that Mrs Wardroper should visit Miss Nightingale more frequently. This we know from notes and correspondence did happen. Miss Nightingale praised Mrs Wardroper's good points and her earnestness, but she continued to find her excitable, tearful, contradictory and unable to express herself with brevity. These visits continued until Mrs Wardroper retired at the age of 74 years.

Another measure that it was hoped would produce an improvement in the standard of training was the appointment of Mr John Croft to organise a more rigorous course of instruction which he did in consultation with the Fund Committee and Miss Nightingale. A syllabus was prepared and a reading list provided, with weekly lectures subsequently printed.[26] The Home sister then held tutorials and improvement classes. Mr Croft's printed lectures are interesting because they indicate the main causes of admission to St Thomas's, showing a strong emphasis on the acute and the cases amenable to the surgery of the day. Although nursing points are emphasised, Mr Croft, like his predecessor, clearly sees his brighter pupils as ancillary doctors able to take over the measuring and treatments previously done by doctors. After 1873 Mr Croft attended the Fund Committee's yearly meetings and henceforth there are fuller reports of the pupils' progress and their examination results. Soon Mr Croft was assisted by Drs Bernays and Peacock, who also submitted reports, and chemistry was added to the curriculum. These reports and letters from probationers show a shift in the duties for probationers. Laura Wilson, writing home to a friend in 1876, tells how she had been taught to use a catheter and dress burns but also relates how she had been upset by the use of human liver for a demonstration at a post-mortem.[27] There are several references to nurses attending autopsies for teaching purposes.

Another probationer to leave a picture of life at St Thomas's in the 1870s was Mary Cadbury, a Quaker, who at the age of 34 years started training as a 'Special Probationer'. Mary wrote home regularly to her mother and her large family in Birmingham, and, with a fine disregard for spelling, punctuation and syntax, she wrote as she felt and from the heart, and fortunately most of these letters have been preserved to give us a Pisgah glimpse of the life in the new St Thomas's in the early 1870s.

First, it is clear that the 'Specials' formed a little coterie within the nursing world; usually coming from similar backgrounds – not needing to earn their living – they saw themselves apart, which is perhaps why Miss Nightingale herself was reluctant to follow the trend of creating an 'officer class'. In spite of the new Nurses' Home, on which so much thought had been lavished, life was Spartan and the group sought solace from one another in their cold bedrooms, with the Nightingale fetish for open windows even on a foggy night. Parcels from home and flowers were shared with one another as they gossiped about their work on the wards, troubles with the nursing hierarchy and their septic fingers, sore throats and the many maladies to which the nineteenth-century nurse was heir. There is an irony in the fact that this was the latest teaching hospital in London and here are nurses treating one another's septic fingers and sore throats with plasters and 'Carrier's' syrup sent by kind Mrs Cadbury from Birmingham. Mary developed a painful boil and also a rash and wrote to her mother, 'Do you think sulphur would do me good?' It is obvious that the many amenities of this imposing edifice did not include a staff treatment room. For relaxation after supper there was sometimes a short walk by the Thames, but the golden circle always seems the same, there is never a mention of socialising with anyone else and this group included three Quakers with whom there was bonding. Mary's only natural activity outside the world of hospital seems to be the occasional visit to the Meeting House, sometimes in the fog, after which she dutifully records the sermon in letters to her mother, interspersed with the events on the wards and accounts of her more lurid cases.

Second, the letters bear out Miss Nightingale's complaint about the lack of a system in allocating probationers and the variable ability of the sisters to teach, or wish to teach. However, Mrs Wardroper had a difficult task; the 'Specials' could, and did, request to stay on, or leave wards. Mary Cadbury asks to stay with Miss Rhodes on Arthur as:

'she could teach me about the murmers of the heart and the sounds of the lungs (sic).'[29]

She declined to go to Victoria because it was 'too hard and worrying'. The Specials obviously developed their own league tables about the sisters', and indeed the doctors', teaching abilities, and it is small wonder that Mrs Wardroper was thought to be 'antagonistic to the Specials'.

Mary tells her mother that she is now on Edward, where the sister is 'a real born lady' and tells you what to do, rather than as happened on her previous ward, where she was left to find out for herself. The preference may have something to do with the ladylike qualities of the sister.[30]

Third, we get a glimpse of Mrs Wardroper as a woman overworked, out of her depth, rather garrulous, a person who does not command respect and who takes refuge in erratic friendships interspersed with bitter antagonisms and one who is probably rather lonely. Mary Cadbury records her initial interview in 1873 when Mrs Wardroper impressed on her that she was 'overwhelmed with applications from ladies', how she never gets to bed until midnight, 'but now Miss Nightingale is helping with the applications which she did not do before'. An indication of Miss Nightingale's somewhat belated interest.

Although Mary Cadbury is not an entirely reliable witness and she suffered from a conflict of purpose, to preach and convert, and to nurse, and we do get a picture of the 'favourites' who came and went. At first Mrs Wardroper was friendly and, according to Mary Cadbury, 'seems to like me' but after 9 months she writes 'Mrs W complains out of the imagination of her heart, or the tittle tattle of the sisters' and 'she distributes her bounty unevenly'.[31] We are left with the impression of intrigue and gossip that is so often the concomitant of a closed community.

The description of life on night duty, after nine months of training, perhaps sheds light on the reason for the high rate of sickness. Writing to mother at 2 am Mary says she must get her 'midnight meal' of bread and butter and tea in the ward kitchen, but she needs to write up her lecture for the next day. At 3.45 am she must prepare the patient's breakfast, which they have at 5 am. At 6 am she starts work, making the beds and presumably leaving the 'Coverlets exactly 6 inches from the floor all round'. She returns to the Home at 8.30 am, a routine with but little modification that was followed for years.

These letters also shed some light on the controversy over the Highgate experiment. Miss Nightingale herself was passionately concerned with the reform of Workhouse nursing, but Mrs Wardroper and some of the Specials were not so keen. Mary Cadbury tried to refuse what was virtually a posting and appealed to Miss Nightingale, apparently in vain. Eventually she goes, reassuring her mother that 'Miss Gregory, Cannon (sic) Gregory's daughter was there last year and said it was good experience. However, she did not enjoy her stay, presumably the already ill Miss Hill was not 'a real born lady' and the patients 'are a much lower class than at St Thomas's. I feel I have come from aristocracy to democracy, nurses, patients and all there is no one that I see to speak to.'[32] She returned to St Thomas's, to her friends, only to cross swords with Mrs Wardroper. She eventually left to join Florence Lees at the Metropolitan and National District Nursing Association in Bloomsbury, a move of which Mrs Wardroper disapproved; like many a later day matron she saw district nursing as a waste of a valuable hospital training.

Mary Cadbury's subsequent career was not always a happy one, she saw it as her Christian duty to put the spiritual needs of her patients before their physical needs and this could lead to conflict with doctors, as it did when she was at Sheffield. There is no doubt but that, like other Victorian ladies justifying their existence by doing unpaid work, she used her position as a means of social control over the lower classes. Miss Nightingale wrote to Mr Rathbone:

> It is most satisfactory to find the Lady Supt and the nurse exercising certain powers and influences in Sanitary matters such as obtaining the cleansing and lime washing of unhealthy houses[33]. Mr Rathbone himself, with his Quaker background, was more concerned about the nurse inspiring temperance.

Another problem arising from the introduction of this 'Special Group' commonly known as Lady Probationers was that just as they had overemphasised the failings of the 'Gamps' before them, they now overemphasised their superior social status: 'If they were not ladies they hoped to be regarded as such.' This was divisive and was an unfortunate legacy for nursing in the twentieth century when 'occupation of father' was of paramount importance on the application form. Among the early 'specials' who survived this rigorous training several did become pioneering superintendents, probably not so much from what they learnt on the wards but what they learnt from one another, and because they were both educated and highly motivated.

In 1874 the Fund Council considered taking drastic action and they sought Counsel's opinion about the Deed of Trust of the Nightingale Fund and Mr Justice Lindley's judgement was submitted to the Committee. The case stated:

> that the objects for which the Fund had been subscribed might best be advanced by a larger expenditure than the income of the Fund would allow and it might be desirable to apply part, or by degrees, the whole of the capital in more rapidly developing the system of training which had been established, and there was no special reason for retaining the Fund

permanently or creating an endowment and the object had been to
support a system which when established would be self-supporting or
continued by the public on account of its intrinsic merit.

On the question as to whether the Trustees would be bound to act on
a request to apply capital Counsel's opinion was

...Miss Nightingale herself has the power to require this to be done and
if she requires it the trustees will, in my opinion be bound to comply. I
doubt whether the Council have like power but this is not necessary to
determine as Miss Nightingale clearly has and she would give written
directions to the trustees... Signed Nath. Lindley, 5 August 1874.[34]

A covering letter from Miss Nightingale suggested that the Council
might apply capital to another School 'with a staff of our own', say in
Edinburgh, Dublin or even Belfast, and that contributions to the
Metropolitan and National Nursing Association be made out of
capital.

The significant suggestion lay in the words 'with a staff of our own'
but from where would such a large staff come – all capable of teaching – and more important, who would have them? The Nightingale
staff would have to displace other staff. There is evidence that there
was a hope that an independent school could be started in Edinburgh,
which once staffed by selected Nightingale nurses would provide a
system for training not only nurses but training future superintendents, a lack at St Thomas's Miss Nightingale constantly bewailed:

There is no training for those who are to train others. Lady Probationers
have no means to qualify themselves for superintendence and training
others which is what we ourselves held out for them...[35]

and

I have said this scores of times, you must be weary of hearing me *we do
not*, to those we expressly hold out the career of superintendence and
training, offer any special training.[36]

In spite of Miss Nightingale's enthusiasm for spending capital, and for
accurately pinpointing the problem with which they needed to deal,
there is no evidence that the Council discussed possible projects, probably for the simple reason that until they had a staff of trainers capital
expenditure on an independent School was of no avail.

In the summer of 1872 an approach was made from the Edinburgh
Royal Infirmary which seemed one way out of the impasse. Edinburgh
wanted a whole staff and there were some thoughts that the School
might be transferred. Miss Barclay was interviewed by the Board in
October and went to Edinburgh in November, from where she sent a

detailed description of the hospital accommodation – or lack of it – and the possibilities of converting the old Fever House for nursing staff. Miss Barclay thought that the Fund should supply nine nurses in the first instance, and her requirements were clear, precise and businesslike.[37] The following staff were selected by the Fund and Mrs Wardroper and sent to Edinburgh: Miss Pringle as assistant and Miss Augusta Lemon, another Special, as Home Sister, Jane Mesher and Margaret Westle as Night Sisters, Eleanor Chisholm and Mary Lyons as Fever Sisters and Ann Monk, Mary Barnard and Victoria Attwood. At the same time, when the accommodation was ready, eight probationers were to be transferred, clear evidence that Edinburgh was intended to be a Nightingale School of Nursing. Like her pioneering colleagues Miss Barclay found many difficulties. In January she was writing:

> I fear there is little chance of success in this most lawless place. Every condition is against us – the inconvenient arrangement of the wards, the surgeon's hours. The head surgeon and the physician tho' expressing themselves anxious to improve the nursing are not willing, when it comes to the point, of giving up their old prerogatives so that my authority is many of the wards is second to theirs and the old nurses are not slow in letting me know it...[38]

However, Mr James Hope, the Secretary to the Governors, expressed himself pleased with Miss Barclay and only hoped that she would not lose heart because there were no answers to her advertisements. As Miss Barclay put it, 'the reputation of the hospital is so bad that only scrubbers apply'.

Mr Bonham Carter urged patience: 'We cannot expect the light to come upon them at once', he wrote, and suggested that Miss Barclay continue with formal contacts with the Committee and informal approaches to the friendly doctors.[39] At the same time there was an interesting confession from Mr Bonham Carter about his difficulty in getting suitable staff from St Thomas's:

> Because the original plan of monthly assessments was never, and never could be, carried out; the various times at which the probationers completed their training rendered it impossible... appointments have been made without my approval because there was no choice.[40]

This was yet a further proof that the Record Book – so beloved by nurse historians as a proof of efficiency – had little value and that it was Mr Bonham Carter who expected to approve appointments.

The first hint that all was not well at Edinburgh was in April when Miss Lemon visited Miss Nightingale and reported on Miss Barclay's health. Miss Nightingale was horrified and wrote to Mr Bonham Carter 'there must be a breakdown before long', though she did not say why. As usual she appealed, 'What's to be done?' They sought advice from Mr Croft and agonised over a successor – 'Pringle was made for a training sister and not for superintendence', 'Williams would do but there was no chance of her recovery for months' – and they were not rich enough to take on Edinburgh and keep St Thomas's 'though some judges (good) think that even as it is Edinburgh is promising'.[41] This may well have been the dilemma that caused Miss Nightingale to seek Counsel's opinion about spending capital.

In spite of Miss Lemon's fears there is an excellent clear letter from Miss Barclay setting out the difficulties which were largely due to the bad name of the hospital, but full of praise for the nurses she had brought with her. She says that she has been giving lectures assisted by Miss Pringle but that she has 'been worried into illness' by the doctors who came into the nurses' rooms at all hours and attended them when they were sick without her knowledge. All, however, appeared in order. There was a printed *System of Training for Edinburgh Royal Infirmary*, modelled on St Thomas's, but with more emphasis on night superintendence and night nursing.

At this stage Miss Nightingale seems more worried about Mrs Wardroper than Miss Barclay:

> My own belief is that Mrs Wardroper is failing so much in mind and body that she will not last six months, but if Miss Pringle comes back she might rally and have a few years longer. But this seems to me the only way out of our overwhelming difficulties at St Thomas's.[42]

Then, in August, Miss Barclay's breakdown seems to have become imminent. Her friends corresponded with Miss Nightingale in secret and this time it looks as if the secret was kept until it could be hushed no longer. In September Miss Nightingale wrote to Mr Bonham Carter on holiday in Stornaway, 'For your eyes alone':

> The end is nearer than we thought – what was seen on that fatal August day has been repeated again and again. She is so little herself that she speaks of determination not to let Pringle remain at Edinburgh... The fatal habit has been one for years!! and they thought we (i.e. I) knew it... The brother Robert is with her now but it is no good. The stimulants used are different. Nurse Mesher is with her and knows all.[43]

Mr Bonham Carter telegraphed 'tell her to resign and that you know everything'.

Miss Barclay, a wreck of a woman addicted to both alcohol and opium, was summoned to Lea Hurst. Miss Nightingale battled for her confession, pledge and redemption; Miss Barclay swore that she was fit to return and in the end, no doubt in order to save a scandal, it was agreed that Miss Barclay should return and stay until November and then either resign on health grounds or ask for six months' leave of absence. When she returned Miss Barclay repudiated her promise and, what was worse, seemed paranoid about Miss Pringle whose removal she was insisting on and who now genuinely wanted to leave. How much the Edinburgh Committee knew is not clear but they acted with great discretion and understanding and gave her leave on health grounds. During her last month Miss Barclay seems to have betrayed signs of real instability, but at the same time made herself as agreeable as possible, boasting that she had the loyalty of the nurses who would see her departure as 'Miss Nightingale's desire and not a matter of her health'. The Committee, anxious to avoid a scandal, arranged for Miss Pringle to act for Miss Barclay and report to her while she was off sick.[44] However, Miss Pringle received such abusive letters that she had to show them to the Committee and eventually the unhappy story closed with Mr Bonham Carter forcing, and quickly accepting, a final resignation. The last ironic twist is a letter from Miss Barclay warning Miss Pringle about accepting drunken nurses.

The episode is interesting inasmuch as it displays a contradictory side of Miss Nightingale. There was not battling for the redemption of Lucy Kidd or others who tried to ease the struggle with drink or drugs. What Miss Pringle, Miss Lemon and other nurses who kept the secret suffered during those eight months can only be imagined, and, as Miss Nightingale said, 'the poissarde scenes that took place at St Thomas's with Mrs Wardroper dragging sisters before Lord Petty Bag [Miss Nightingale's nickname for Mr Baggallay] their faults were virtues compared with this'.[45]

Miss Barclay's resignation altered all ideas about bringing in Miss Pringle to watch over Mrs Wardroper. Miss Pringle, 'unfit for super-intendence' supported by 'unfit' Miss Williams, had to remain in Edinburgh. In the event they worked well together, were much liked by the Committee and eventually won over the doctors. In her 14 years at Edinburgh Miss Pringle ran a successful training school with limited resources and trained many matrons for their schools. When Miss Williams left in 1876 she was replaced by Frances Spencer, another of that outstanding group of Specials who trained between 1870 and 1872, and who remained friends. By 1882 the Edinburgh School could boast 38 probationers, four courses of doctors' lectures a year, classes held by the Home sister and a course of lectures given by the Edinburgh School of Domestic Science. As the result of its success Edinburgh could now largely fill its own vacancies and was at the same time supplying head nurses to other hospitals in Scotland.

During the mid-1870s when the Fund was looking for an alternative to St Thomas's, or some means of putting their eggs in different baskets, it is important to differentiate between the schemes where the Fund actually had financial arrangements and hospitals where they sent a group of nurses, because vacancies were advertised, and in the hope that they would persuade the governors to start a training scheme without money from the Fund. Money had been invested in the School at Highgate and when that closed, a few years later, a similar arrangement was made with St Marylebone. Now, once the School in Edinburgh was running successfully, the Fund looked around for another London voluntary hospital. In 1875 a request came from the Board of Governors of St Mary's Hospital, Paddington, which seems to have arisen out of the survey by Miss Florence Lees in 1874[46] which gives a concise picture of St Mary's at that time. There were only 160 beds with the wards opening on to one another where the Registrar was responsible for the ventilation. Miss Wright, the matron, had no training and did not have the power to engage or dismiss the nursing staff, who consisted of six sisters, six ward nurses, seven night nurses and six assistants; the staff slept in dormitories and had no bathroom or day room. These were some of the things that had to be rectified before the Fund Council would entertain the idea of co-operating and sending a team of nurses.

After considerable correspondence it was decided to advise Rachel Williams from Edinburgh to apply for the post of Lady Superintendent. She was successful out of 32 candidates and took up her duties in October 1876. But between her appointment and taking up her duties it is clear that Miss Williams had qualms, and like so many of her contemporaries her great fear was about the night nursing and the 'general lawlessness at night'.[47] Problems with the night staff, however, were nothing compared with the usual problem of Nightingale superintendents, that of carving out an empire and a definite sphere of influence. There was trouble with the steward who controlled the kitchen and the standard of cleanliness, and, in spite of the fact that Miss Williams had taken with her Miss Enderby as her assistant and seven other Nightingales, the first years were far from easy. In 1877 Miss Williams had cause to dismiss a sister whose case was taken up by a Dr Broadbent who laid complaints before the Committee about Miss Williams. This led to a complicated enquiry with a report drawn up by Sir Thomas Pycroft. Miss Williams, duly briefed and supported by Mr Bonham Carter, appeared before the Committee and after several unsatisfactory meetings a compromise was eventually reached. Miss Williams remained and the sister went.[48] Once again the row had been about accountability and the power of the matron to engage and dismiss nursing staff. Rachel Williams was an outspoken Quaker and although Miss Nightingale called her the Goddess because of her beauty and willowy height, she was apparently far from angelic in temperament; in spite of her sentimental letters Miss Nightingale sometimes dreaded her visits. At St Mary's the Goddess met the Greeks in the form of the doctors and her tenure of office seems to have been marked by passages of arms.

Although Miss Williams had 16 probationers in 1880, according to Zachary Cope there was no training school with lectures until 1885 when Miss Medill from the Middlesex took over.[49] The last few years were unhappy for Miss Williams, she often spoke of leaving, and there was an unseemly dispute about her salary in which she behaved with great dignity. Again Dr Broadbent led the attack and eventually the Committee, while exonerating Miss Williams, asked for her resignation – a request that coincided with her own wish to leave – and she handed in her resignation on 23 January 1885. Fortunately she was almost immediately asked by the government to lead a band of nurses in the Egyptian campaign after which she married Mr Daniel Norris. Later she became the superintendent of a Nursing Home in Cannes, where she died in 1908. *Facilis descensus Averni.* The object of the valuable Nightingale training was to give better nursing to the sick poor in hospitals and on the district. It is surprising how many Nightingale nurses ended their careers running nursing homes for profit.

Nightingale nurses obtained the superintendence of two other London voluntary hospitals – St Bartholomew's and the Westminster. According to Miss Lees' report in 1875 the nursing at St Bartholomew's was still unreformed with no attempt at a training system. In 1877 it seems that Mr Bonham Carter persuaded Sir Sydney Waterlow, chairman of the governors, whom he knew in connection with the Poor Law, to advertise for a Lady Superintendent and make arrangements for a Nurses' Home and for probationers who would receive lectures from Mr Dyce Duckworth. At first it was thought that Miss Solly would apply but, when in that summer Miss Machin and her team returned from Canada, protracted negotiations were started for her appointment. After frustrating delays Miss Machin, with Helen Blower as her assistant, sisters Jane Styring and Ann Fryer and nurses Robinson, Gardner, Parr, Trueman and Wilson went to St Bartholomew's in November 1878.

A tentative 'school' was opened in 1877 and Miss Machin lengthened the training to two years, but in spite of the close relationship of the governors and the Fund Miss Machin does not seem to have been happy at St Bartholomew's though it is not clear why, and after some dispute she resigned in 1880. When Ethel Manson, aged 25 years, from the London Hospital, arrived as the superintendent in 1881 the Nightingale influence at St Bartholomew's was virtually at an end. Miss Manson started a three-year training and a philosophy to training that was largely antagonistic to that of Miss Nightingale.

The situation at the Westminster and its sister hospital, St George's, was different. With Lady Augusta Stanley, wife of Dean Stanley, on the Board there was an early active interest in nursing.[50] In the 1860s, with a view to improving the nursing, the Board examined the various systems of nursing in practice; these included the St John's sisterhood and the Liverpool system where the Lady Superintendent engaged nurses and supplied them to a hospital for a fixed sum; this was judged to be the most economical and the two Miss Merryweathers were persuaded to come to Westminster, Mary as Lady Superintendent and Elizabeth, her sister, as matron. They started a training school in 1873 but the division of duties did not work and there were disagreements between the Merryweathers and the Committee. When Mary died Elizabeth left and the governors resolved to combine the two posts on the Nightingale pattern. Miss Lees had reported that under the Merryweathers there was no systematic plan of training, the same complaint as was levelled at the Liverpool Royal Hospital. When Miss Pyne, a Nightingale Fund nurse, took over the superintendence in 1880 it was an assessment with which she did not disagree. Miss Pyne remained at the Westminster, apparently successfully, until 1898.

By 1882 there were Nightingale Fund nurses as matrons at the following hospitals: the Sydney Hospital, New South Wales; Royal Victoria Hospital, Netley; Edinburgh Royal Infirmary; St Mary's Hospital, London; the Westminster Hospital, London; Liverpool Royal Infirmary; the Southern Hospital, Liverpool; St Marylebone Workhouse Infirmary; Salisbury Infirmary; Lincoln Infirmary; Leeds Infirmary; Huntingdon County Hospital; Cumberland Infirmary and the Royal Hospital for Incurables, Putney.[51]

After this period, however, the Fund's share in the number of superintendent posts in large hospitals began to fall because other hospitals had also been running training schools with Lady Probationers, and the products of these were also applying for, and taking, top posts. Nevertheless, in spite of the difficulties and the setbacks the Fund had captured a high proportion of the commanding heights of nursing and had in each case established the matron as supreme in nursing matters.

Notes

1. Sir James Clark to FN, GLRO, HI/ST/NC2/V25/67, 9 August 1867.
2. Lambert, R., *Sir John Simon 1816–1904* (MacGibbon & Kee, London, 1963), p. 482.
3. *The Nightingale Fund Council Report* (Year ending 25 December 1871), para 3.
4. Parsons, F., *The History of St. Thomas's Hospital* (Methuen, London, 1936), vol. 3.
5. *The Lancet*, 31 March 1866; also *Pall Mall Magazine* (February 1866) (see also Chapter 3).
6. FN to H. Bonham Carter, BL, Add Mss 47717, 29 November 1872, f. 120.
7. E. Rappe to FN, BL, Add Mss 47759, June 1867, f. 217.
8. FN to H. Bonham Carter (quoting E. Torrance), BL, Add Mss 47716, 24 November 1871, f. 202.
9. FN to H. Bonham Carter, GLRO, HI/ST/NC1/72, 12, 18 May 1872.
10. H. Bonham Carter to FN, GLRO, HI/ST/V13/71, July 1871.
11. H. Bonham Carter to FN, GLRO, HI/ST/V3/72, 2 February 1872.
12. Printed Statement on Nursing at the Middlesex Hospital, BL, Add Mss 45752, June 1865–6, f. 125. See also Middlesex Hospital Records Minutes 1866.
13. H. Bonham Carter to FN, GLRO, HI/ST/V3/72, 2 February 1872.
14. GLRO, HI/ST/NC1/72 12a, 18 May 1872.
15. FN to H. Bonham Carter, GLRO, HI/ST/NC1/72/49, November 1872.
16. FN to H. Bonham Carter, GLRO, HI/ST/NC1/72, 12a, June 1872.
17. Ibid., Part 2.
18. R. Whitfield to FN, GLRO, HI/NC1/72, 27, June 1872.
19. H. Bonham Carter to FN, GLRO, HI/ST/NC2/V57/72, November 1872.
20. FN to J. Sutherland, BL, Add Mss 47742, June 1872, f. 238.
21. Minutes of the Nightingale Fund Committee May 1873, GLRO, ANC/A/21.
22. FN to H. Bonham Carter, GLRO, HI/ST/NC1/72 16, 10 June 1872.
23. FN to H. Bonham Carter, GLRO, HI/ST/NC1/72, 8 November 1872.
24. FN to H. Bonham Carter, GLRO, HI/ST/NC1/72, 57, November 1872.
25. H. Bonham Carter to FN, GLRO/ HI/ST/NC1/72, 49, November 1872.
26. Croft, J., *Notes of Lectures* (Blades, East & Blades, London, 1874).
27. Laura Wilson to 'Anne', GLRO, HI/ST/NTS/Y17, 13 May 1876.
28. GLRO HI/ST/NTS/Y16/2, Letter 18 March 187#.
29. GLRO HI/ST/NTS/Y16/2, Letter, 5 July 1873.
30. GLRO HI/ST/NTS/Y16/2, Letter, 15 March 1874.
31. GLRO HI/ST/NTS/Y16/2, Letter, 18 March 1874.
32. GLRO HI/ST/NTS/Y16/2, Letter, 19 ?March 1974.
33. Nightingale, F,. Introduction to the *Organisation of Nursing in a Large Town:*, Rathbone, Wm. (Longman, Green, London, 1865) (quoted in Baly, *History of the Queen's Institute*, Croom Helm, London, 1986).
34. Minutes of the Nightingale Fund Committee March 1876, together with

covering letter from FN, GLRO, A/NFC/2/1.

35 FN to H. Bonham Carter, BL, Add Mss 47717, 1 February 1873, f. 216.

36. FN to H. Bonham Carter, BL, Add Mss 47719, 21 October 1876, f. 170.

37. E. Barclay to S. Wardroper, BL, Add Mss 47719, 14 October 1872, f. 87.

38. E. Barclay to H. Bonham Carter, BL, Add Mss 47719, 7 January 1873, f. 162.

39. H. Bonham Carter to E. Barclay, BL, Add Mss 47718, 14 March 1873, f. 4.

40. H. Bonham Carter to James Hope, BL, Add Mss 47718, 14 March 1873, f. 3.

41. FN to H. Bonham Carter, BL, Add Mss 47718, 8 April 1873, f. 47.

42. FN to H. Bonham Carter, BL, Add Mss 47718, 4 July 1873, f. 135.

43. FN to H. Bonham Carter, BL, Add Mss 47718, 22 September 1873, f. 188 and f. 190.

44. H. Bonham Carter to FN, BL, Add Mss 47718, 17 November 1873, f. 253.

45. FN to H. Bonham Carter, BL, Add Mss 47718, October 1873, f. 200.

46. Miss Lees' Survey of London Hospitals, GLRO, A/NFC/22/2.

47. R. Williams to H. Bonham Carter, GLRO, HI/ST/NC18/12, 14 & 15, 13 July 1876.

48. Dr Sieveking to H. Bonham Carter, GLRO, HI/ST/NC18.12, 5, 7 & 19 May 1877.

49. Cope, Z., *A Hundred Years of Nursing at St. Mary's Paddington* (Heinemann, London, 1955), Chapter V.

50. Humble, J.G. and Hansell, P., *The Westminster 1716–1974* (Pitman Medical, London, 1974).

51. *The Nightingale Fund Council Annual Report*, 1882.

10. The Nightingale Training School 1875–1890

> As we are I am not sure that the hard drive of the probationers is a bad thing. At least it knocks the ministering angel nonsense out of their heads and makes them look at nursing as the urgent business like work it really is. But then it knocks something else too out of their heads – to wit goodness and all high aspiration.
>
> *Florence Nightingale, 17 January 1873*

The Fund Council did not spend capital, instead it relied on a pragmatic approach to its many problems. Money would not buy what was needed which was sufficient numbers of trained, educated sisters who were capable of teaching and who had time to teach, and a system of regular classroom instruction. Miss Nightingale put her finger on the nub of the problem when she said:

> If we had experienced sisters, if we had a matron with any system, if we had a Head to the Home, most certainly with 33–35 probationers to 330 beds, at least two hours a day – besides proper rest and exercise, could be spared for each probationer for classes.[1]

But after 13 years the Fund had none of these things. 'We were the making of St Thomas's, St Thomas's now truly is the unmaking of us', bemoaned Miss Nightingale,[2] but who else could be the making of them? Even if a scheme could be devised – and paid for – whereby the probationers were truly supernumerary, who would teach them? The Fund Council did the only thing it could do and that was to try and improve the situation at St Thomas's and hope that eventually there would be experienced teaching sisters and a new understanding of the probationers' educational needs.

The mainstay of the new approach was the Home sister, but three had come and gone in quick succession, and in 1875 Mary Crossland took over this unenviable task. Miss Crossland was a clergyman's daughter who had been a governess before coming to St Thomas's and although she sometimes expressed a desire to leave she did stay until her retirement, fortified by a strong belief that it was her Christian duty and close contact with Miss Nightingale. Miss Crossland was a frequent visitor to South Street reporting to Miss Nightingale on a wide range of topics including the teaching abilities – or otherwise – of the sisters and the state of nursing in the hospital. Miss Nightingale kept notes of these interviews and from these and the correspondence we get a picture of the nursing and the progress of the School.

The tripod of nurse training was to be the ward instruction, doctor's lectures backed by the Home sister's tuition in both nursing and moral matters, and the taking of case notes and the keeping of diaries. In practice each leg of the tripod was weak but perhaps the weakest was ward teaching. With rare exceptions the ward sisters had neither the time nor the ability to teach, and even the Lady Probationers trained under the Fund were deficient in this respect because their training was task-orientated without supervision and they were not taught to teach others. As Miss Nightingale complained:

> You train ladies in the express principle that they are leaders of their own nurses yet what means do you give them of doing this most desirable thing? She [sic] receives exactly the same training as the nurses (none receives any scientific training). No opportunity is given to any of them to learn what you profess they ought to do.[31]

One way out of this difficulty would have been for the Home sister to have given clinical instruction on the wards and for the probationers to have had two hours in the classroom each day, but the first Mrs Wardroper forbade and the second she could not organise because the probationers were ward assistants. Miss Nightingale found this 'cutting off very objectionable' and she thought that from 'time to time the Home Sister should communicate with the ward sisters about probationers she may feel uneasy about' but this Mrs Wardroper would not allow.[4] Class teaching and ward teaching were destined to remain separate.

One likely reason why Mrs Wardroper was reluctant to allow the Home sister on to the wards to give instruction was the attitude of the doctors. Not all the doctors welcomed the reformed nursing system. Mr Whitfield, for example, was probably reflecting his colleagues when he said that teaching probationers about case histories was objectionable. Under the old system the sister was accountable to the doctor, who taught her enough to carry out *his* orders, and there was appropriate male domination of women's work – 'the old nurse was eminently deferential... there was never any doubt as to who was the master'.[5]

Now there was doubt; the Lady Superintendent decided what should be taught and when, the nurses were to be moved according to their training needs, which the doctors resented – as some saw this as conflicting with the training needs of medical students. To have introduced another woman to the wards, not accountable to them, teaching what they often described as 'quackery' would have been a further irritant and Mrs Wardroper was no doubt merely keeping the peace. Nursing as noble and womanly work was one thing, but teaching them to reason why was another; this invited questioning and was a challenge to medical power. Well might Henry Bonham Carter write:

> He [the doctor] thinks his telling the nurse what she ought to do is nearly enough to perfect her... he requires to be told more distinctly than ever why this is not enough and that no training can be sufficient where he is the principal.[6]

The doctors' lectures after 1874 were certainly an improvement on the almost complete lack before, but neither the lecturers nor the hearers seemed to be clear about the level of understanding that was required or expected. Mr Croft's lectures were useful but they were a strange amalgam of what has been described as 'cook book' nursing, such as the precise way to make a linseed or bread poultice,[7] and material suitable for junior medical students. It is interesting to note that Miss Nightingale who earlier had been so fearful of nurses becoming 'medical women' and who had complained that Mr Whitfield's early lectures were for medical students only, some 15 years later, and after ten years of special probationers, wrote off Mr Croft's lectures:

> Mr Croft's lectures are excellent, but are of the most elementary nature and strictly for nurses. (We shall have our Lady P's going elsewhere to get knowledge for there is scarcely a good school that does not give them more than we do.)[8]

Miss Nightingale was nothing if not inconsistent. The comment, however, highlights the changing demands of medicine in the space of some 20 years and the new expectations for knowledge of educated women.

Miss Nightingale and the Fund Council were soon to find that 'Educating the lady with her cook' posed problems. Apart from being unsure as to the subject matter they ought to impart, the lecturers were confused about the level of understanding of their pupils. Mr Croft wrote: 'A considerable number of the probationers were not capable of writing with sufficient fluency to keep up with the lecturer... the names of those who made notes are attached.'[9]

As time went by the weak were weeded out by examinations and testing, but the lecturer's comments continue to imply that the level of intelligence and the background of education was wide, probably too wide to allow purely theoretical instruction to be meaningful. Nor was Miss Crossland's level of expectation high. Of Dr Bernays' lectures she wrote that they were 'so clear and simple that all enter in and enjoy them, and then he dictates short axioms for them to write down, kindly spelling the hard words and not forgetting the punctuations'.[10] Dr Peacock not only lectured, he also supervised the note taking, but like his colleagues he commented on the wide range of ability of the young ladies. On Dr Bristowe there is the splendid comment that he forgot his notes and presented 'An immense amount of matter to our minds in a more or less confused state and our weak female minds cannot digest or profit by such teaching.'[11] History does not relate what Miss Nightingale thought about 'weak female minds'.

Two main problems dogged the Fund's training scheme then, and for the next century. First, with medicine advancing rapidly and becoming more scientific, no one, not even Miss Nightingale, was sure what was the proper task of the nurse especially within the limited sphere of the acute general hospital. Well had she written, 'I use the word nursing for want of a better'.[12] The probationers were taking on more tasks like testing urine but was that nursing? Related to the first problem was the second: what was the level of intelligence, background education and training needed to meet that proper task? The Nightingale Fund had started by appealing to artisan's daughters and working-class women to whom it offered a worthy and respectable method of earning a living. But this class did not produce leaders and teachers and, somewhat hesitantly, the Fund shifted its appeal to the better educated, and when it needed the money, to those who could afford to pay for their own keep. The classes the lecturers faced had a wide range of general education, this we know from the lecture notes and examination papers that survive, but even more so from the letters the probationers wrote many of which, from all groups, are preserved. There is no doubt that some of the Special Probationers wrote with assurance, fluency and knowledge that betokened real leadership calibre, these were women who would have no difficulty in commanding others. There are, however, a wide range of quite adequate, respectful but well-phrased letters, often to Mr Bonham Carter, from ordinary probationers which indicate that in spite of the lack of formal educational facilities most women could express themselves on paper. However from Miss Crossland's comments there must have been a minority who were almost illiterate, and they of course did not leave letters for the archives. Usually such left their training with the comment 'felt their want of education' but we know also from the comments of some superintendents that a few slipped through the net and were sent out as Nightingale trained nurses.

The lecturers therefore did the best they could in the short time they had with their hard-worked pupils who, according to Miss Nightingale, fell asleep once they were able to sit down. Those who were keen and intelligent supplemented their studies by reading and, as Miss Nightingale surmised, by borrowing from doctor friends either at home or in the hospital. Often, however, as she also rightly surmised, it was undirected study. Reading lists show that the only books advised were medical books and thus the medical model was reinforced: 'The stupid ones read and are puffed up and don't understand. The clever ones understand enough to know that they don't understand and are discouraged having no one to answer their questions.'[13]

The third leg of the training tripod was the Report book and the keeping of diaries and case notes. Once Miss Nightingale started seeing the probationers, she then sent for the Red Register with its 14 headings and compared the official entries with her own notes, hence the red pencil remarks in Register Book B, which began in 1871.[14] Perhaps the most startling of Miss Nightingale's comments was on a young lady who had more than the usual share of 'goods' in the various columns: 'Queer and rough. Quite unfit for children. If I were a patient I would not have her in a mile of me.'

Of one woman Mrs Wardroper wrote 'is likely to be a good nurse'; Miss Nightingale wrote: 'deficient in truth, management and steadiness, a coarse low sort of woman but with capabilities which had she a stricter probation would have made her a more successful nurse and a better woman'.

A young lady of 24 years who had a string of 'moderates' had this in red pencil on her page: 'a very moderate woman indeed: moderate in principles and steadiness. Not to be trusted in a General hospital for her own sake: light in her conduct with men. Not moderated flippancy and impropriety.' As the nurse in question had a good report, one wonders from where Miss Nightingale got her information, possibly of course from Miss Crossland or one of the sisters whose views on probationers did not coincide with those of Mrs Wardroper. But not all the remarks were condemnatory; some gave praise: 'a very strong feeling for her work and the love of it nurse-y and acceptable to her patients. A good little woman.' One thing seems fairly certain: the red pencil would not agree with Mrs Wardroper's assessments.

Next Miss Nightingale's eagle eye fell on the diaries. She was critical of the time spent on routine work, for example, 'the pinning up of checks [quilts] takes a ridiculous time',[15] and in the same note she said 'this can hardly be called training'. And in a comment that was to be re-echoed by reformers for the next hundred years,

> These are the horaries not of probationers but of ward assistants. We do not glean from these at all what they are doing in their special position of learning, or what is being done by way of teaching... sister scarcely appears at all... the diaries are interesting as giving some account of the menial and dressing work but they afford not the slightest clue to what the place is doing as a training school.[16]

The diaries that are preserved, which are mainly from the Special Probationers, are invaluable because they show what the routine was like and what the nurses were doing on a hospital ward in the last quarter of the nineteenth century. Sometimes a few terse entries evoke a picture of the evening in the ward by gaslight and of the patients being settled for the night, not with sedatives but by brandy and wine, as the weary probationers arranged the ink stands, took out the flowerpots, lighted the lamps and finally came off duty to their prayers. The diary in the Appendix is as late as 1890 and shows that even then the Lady Probationer in question was on duty on the ward for ten hours and during her three and a half hours off she attended a lecture. The diaries also show, what was to be shown by job analysis some 60 years later, that most of the probationer's day was unsupervised.[17]

Since Miss Nightingale was given to exaggeration, it is difficult to assess whether the official reports or the red pencil comments are the more accurate. One tentative way is to follow up the more glaring discrepancies and see what happened to those who received good reports from Mrs Wardroper but adverse comments from Miss Nightingale. Some of Miss Nightingale's own swans turned out to be geese, like Miss Barclay, although of course, in some cases, her good report may have been a self-fulfilling prophesy. On the other hand, Mrs Wardroper's judgements do seem to be haphazard in the extreme and some of her favourite like Martin, Duke and Butler did really turn out to be black sheep. An unexpectedly high number in both categories married, often in their late thirties, and these, like the immoderate young lady, are lost to nursing and further analysis.

One can only guess how Mrs Wardroper reacted to the red pencil on her report book, and indeed on her own reports. With the advent of the Lady Probationers her position was becoming more difficult. Miss Nightingale wrote:

> I think Mrs W discourages the lady candidates for two reasons
>
> 1. She and the treasurer wish at least half the work to be done by our probationers.
> 2. She is afraid of the ladies and distrusts her power of managing them.[18]

Contrary to popular belief Miss Nightingale regarded Mrs Wardroper as 'lacking in education', but of course Mrs Wardroper had struggled as a widow with a young family, was not a nurse and did not pretend to be one. As the doctors and their more scientific lectures grew more esoteric and the ladies grew younger while she grew older, now into her late sixties, she must have felt more and more excluded. The social divide was not confined to Miss Nightingale and Mrs Wardroper. Mr Bonham Carter thought that the treasurer was the root of much of the trouble 'because he was not a gentleman'. In all the difficulties between the Fund and the officials of St Thomas's there is the feeling of a certain class distinction.

1878 seems to have been a crisis year. A report on the sanitary state of St Thomas's hospital revealed that the new building was far from hygienic. In this most expensive-to-run hospital, windows were difficult to open, chutes for soiled linen were not used, buckets were without lids, lifts were not used because they took so long and chamber pots were left under beds hidden by the pinned-down quilts. The sharpest criticism was reserved for night duty: it was the only hospital where the night staff came on duty without a meal or did not have one on going off. Moreover, there was no one to see that the night staff kept regular hours of sleep and exercise and there were no classes for night staff; the night nurses were too young to carry so much responsibility without supervision and they were often sick because of the foul air. These criticisms about night duty make interesting reading because some, particularly those about the lack of supervision and proper meals, were still being made at the beginning of the National Health Service.[19]

This report, especially the comments on night duty, is largely borne out by correspondence from Miss Crossland who was now hoping to be transferred to Edinburgh, and who wrote to Miss Nightingale, 'I have long had a desire to work in Edinburgh under Miss Pringle; it is very trying at times working under a failing head.'[20] Miss Crossland was persuaded to stay and continued, as she put it, 'grinding' her pupils and sending Miss Nightingale suggestions for her addresses to the probationers and accounts of the Sunday service.

Another reason for believing that the report on the sanitary state of the hospital was not exaggerated was the fact that the sickness rate remained high. For example, in 1880 39 probationers were recruited of whom 14 were Specials and 16 resigned or were dismissed, but the overriding reason for departure in all classes was ill health. The figures and wastage, particularly on health grounds, in the neighbouring years were much the same. Continuing ill health among the nurses was the reason for Mr Bonham Carter, in conjunction with Mr Croft, issuing the *Memorandum for Probationers*.[21] This is a leaflet with 17 instructions about preventative measures and self-care, particularly with a view to avoiding that scourge of nurses, the septic finger. Much reliance is placed on carbolic soap and oil, and it is interesting to note that 'no nurse should eat or drink until she had changed the apron and oversleeves she has worn on the ward'. And, with a nod to the miasma theory, 'when you have been breathing foul air, you are recommended to ask immediate advice on the subject from the ward sister'. However, in spite of Miss Nightingale's correct assessment that most of the ill health was preventable, other hospitals of the same period had the same story of woe which was not mitigated until aseptic techniques and barrier nursing for infections were properly established.

Apart from the problem of sickness Miss Nightingale was increasingly disturbed about the poor relationship between the Home and hospital, and the fact that Miss Crossland was not allowed on the wards. In June 1878 she wrote:

> I feel we cannot go on after October at St Thomas's without some examination or test as to how the training is conducted. Ought we to go on giving the sisters gratuities for the training without some knowledge of our own...We put these particulars on our list of duties, print them on our sister's records and then have not the least idea, and Mrs Wardroper still less, of how they are carried out, or not carried out.[22]

In August Mr Bonham Carter put an end to the training for six months. 'There are strong indications of great defects', he wrote, the main defect being that between five wards there were two trained nurses and 20 probationers and the two trained nurses had been engaged without consultation with the Fund. It is difficult to trace this hiatus in training in the record books because of the lack of an ordered intake, but the following March when admissions resumed the Fund Committee agreed 'to afford some means of training in the duties of supervision' and Mr Bonham Carter was authorised to make arrangements for selected probationers to receive instruction from the night superintendent 'provided a competent person be appointed'.[23] However, the minutes show that the following year no such an appointment had been made and the Committee, in desperation, decided to authorise a scheme whereby a Lady Probationer, after completing her course at St Thomas's, should be sent to Edinburgh 'to receive instructions in the duties of supervision'. At a meeting of the Committee, yet a year later, it was recorded that 'no opportunity had arisen to implement the scheme'.[24]

Mrs Wardroper had failed to make the necessary arrangements. Periodically the Fund Committee continued to raise the question of the need for a longer, and different training, for superintendence, but for some reason or another it was always deemed to be 'not practical at that time'. About the same time, in the autumn of 1881, there appeared in *The Queen* a strong criticism of the Fund. The journalist had read the Reports of the Fund and had calculated that:

> In the 20 years the school had been open 604 probationers had been admitted of whom only 357 had completed their allotted period of one year's training and entered on the duties of the situations to which they were appointed.

The article goes on to point out that the cost of training worked out at £80 for each probationer and expenditure had exceeded income by £100. Rubbing salt into the wound it goes on:

> Either persons wholly unfitted for their proposed duties have been selected in the first instance, who afterwards have to be discharged; or the regulation must be so irksome, and the duties so arduous, that probationers resign of their own accord thus entailing a useless and unprofitable employment of the income of the Fund.
>
> In no other organisation for special instruction or training for special service are we aware of a similar condition of things. In training colleges for public teachers a very small percentage covers the loss of rejected candidates.

The article then looks at the contract of service and the despotic power given to the matron and finds both likely to conduce resignation. Not unreasonably the journalist confused the Council, 'Eight gentlemen the majority of whom hold official positions that would of necessity prevent them taking a very active personal part in the control of the school and its inmates', and the Committee, which by now was the same as the Council, but which was not clear in the official reports. 'Officers', the article complained, were 'not named but the Secretary'. But of course the secretary was, to all intents and purposes, the only person besides Miss Nightingale who really mattered. Nor did the journalist realise the close kinship and personal relationship between some members of the Committee which made informal communication possible:

> With every sympathy for the education and training of nurses we cannot imagine a system which centralises the power of selection and instantaneous dismissal without any reason being alleged, in the hands of one lady, is calculated to work advantageously.

The article concludes with an exhortation for 'A little more sunshine in the lives of these young women'.[25] In many ways the Fund Council could not disagree. The article highlighted the problem that they had made for themselves, though with some dissenting voices – the 'despotic power' given to the matron. Even before the article there were doubts; Henry Bonham Carter thought that it was a disincentive to recruitment and in 1878 Miss Nightingale had written:

> My views are exceedingly altered as to the supremacy of the matron. It did very well for me whose fault is subserviency and civility. It does ill for matrons whose fault is the lover of power and lawlessness towards medical and other authorities and for matronships where there is not strong and intelligent administration with power and duties running parallel to the matrons.[26]

Miss Nightingale's views may have altered, but the die was cast. The Fund had fought to ensure that the matron was supreme, and supreme she would remain. Nor did Miss Nightingale's views revert once Mrs Wardroper had left. In 1894, during Miss Gordon's matronship, Miss Nightingale wrote:

> I am not so sure that the nursing ought to be so entirely in the matron's hands now. We have no dominance over her now. We have recommended people lately who ought not to be in a mile of the hospital.[27]

But by now the nursing administration had carved out and consolidated its empire. Later, in any attempt to emasculate it, it perversely evoked that early authority of Miss Nightingale. Nursing not only gave women a respectable job, it gave some a career structure with opportunities for authority and power in a world where such opportunities were few.

In considering the criticism of *The Queen's* magazine it must be remembered that the simple arrangement drawn up by the Fund in 1860 was for working-class women who had to be seen to be under strict discipline, for it was this discipline and moral respectability that marked off the experiment from what had gone before. The matron was given so much power because she had to enforce discipline, and it was judged, probably rightly, that she would do it more thoroughly than those who had attempted the task before. Now, however, Miss Nightingale was hoist with her own petard. Twenty years had seen changes in attitudes to women at work and their working conditions; women, albeit with much opposition, were entering medicine, there were more choices, and women's education, women's rights and trade unions were all making their mark. By 1890 despotic rule and dismissal without reason were frowned upon – especially for the newly educated middle classes who were now forming a proportion of the Nightingale ladies. The criticism was made worse by the discovery that Mrs Wardroper received over 1,000 applications in 1883, from which she selected 19 of whom ten survived their training, and in her last year 24 were selected from 1,455 candidates.[28] How many of the applications were totally unsuitable it is difficult to say but obviously by 1885 the high wastage figure could not be laid at the door of no choice.

In spite of the criticisms little was done, or could be done, to alter the fundamental set-up. After 1882 Mrs Wardroper's reports became fuller, she had a clerk, possibly one of her sons, and there is more emphasis on the character of the sisters and on ward teaching. It also began to look as if the closing of the school had a salutary effect.

However, there was little improvement either in the sanitary condition of the hospital or the Home, a fact which was adversely commented on by the London Sanitary Protection Society.[29] The same year, 1885, Mrs Wardroper, now over 70 years old, reported that the sickness rate had been exceptional and that the probationers were ill due to defects in the Home itself. For the previous year she reported that 26 candidates out of 40 had either resigned or been dismissed, and again the main reason was either ill health or unsuitable behaviour. The illness was such that the training pattern was disrupted and classes abandoned.

In 1886, when it was known that Mrs Wardroper would retire, the Fund Council prepared a special report in the form of a 15-page booklet to mark their achievements.[30] The cracks and the disputes are papered over in Henry Bonham Carter's most tactful style, though what is left unsaid is as important as what is said. There is, for example, no comment on the analysis of entries to the school for the year in question. Of the 47 probationers admitted 23 had resigned or been dismissed. Of those who completed their training 15 went on to the staff of St Thomas's and the remainder to associated hospitals and the Metropolitan and National Nursing Association. St Thomas's and its associates were now absorbing most of the trainees.

The printed survey of what the Fund had achieved was impressive. Miss Nightingale was not allowed to spoil the laudatory tone by erasing names like Miss Osburn, or the name of Mrs Deeble as the Superintendent of Netley. The report sets out the experiments with which the Fund had been associated and the Schools it had started, namely, the Highgate Infirmary, the Royal Infirmary, Edinburgh, St Marylebone Infirmary, St Mary's Paddington and the Metropolitan and National Nursing Association, all of which, with the exception of the last, had turned, or were turning out, 'Nightingale' nurses. St Thomas's was now the mother house, not only for nurses scattered across the world, but also for whole training schools. Having listed the

hospitals to which Nightingale nurses had been sent as superintendents the report goes on to refer to Mrs Wardroper's retirement and
to state that

> The object for which the school was established has been obtained grad-
> ually, quietly and without ostentation, with perfect harmony on all sides;
> this success has been largely due to the matron, Mrs Wardroper.

Tact and public propaganda could hardly go further.

Sir William Bowman read Miss Nightingale's address to the probationers; he was followed by Mr William Rathbone who read the panegyric to Mrs Wardroper. All the social niceties were preserved and
Mrs Wardroper was presented with a tea service and a pension of
£100 a year from the Fund.

It is difficult to know what Miss Nightingale's and Mr Bonham
Carter's true feelings were on Mrs Wardroper's retirement. There is
no evidence in the letters that they did not find her a stumbling block
to their plans to the bitter end. Nevertheless Miss Nightingale, in spite
of being downright libellous with her pen dipped in gall, seems to have
had a certain affection for this old lady, who, in spite of her faults, had
'great qualities' and who remained loyal to the Fund, often making
long journeys on its behalf. One senses that in spite of being irritated
by her incoherent thought, Miss Nightingale was sorry for
Mrs Wardroper and was continually urging herself to be more chari-
table. After an outburst about Mrs Wardroper's indecision to Rachel
Williams she wrote:

> Teach me to feel another's woe,
> To hide the fault I see
> That I mercy to others show
> That mercy show to me.[31]

When Mrs Wardroper died in 1892 Miss Nightingale wrote the
much quoted 'A Nursing Worthy' for the *Hospital Nursing
Supplement*[32] in which she refers to Mrs Wardroper's hard life and to
the fact that 'she never went a-pleasuring'. Her highest praise was 'her
judgement of character came by intuition' which was a kind
euphemism for what she had written so many times about Mrs
Wardroper's judgement of character being nil.

After Mrs Wardroper's retirement Miss Pringle at last returned to
St Thomas's as the Lady Superintendent and the matron of the hospital. Both Mr Bonham Carter and Miss Nightingale were delighted. Of
all the Nightingale nurses the 'Pearl' was the most universally admired;
she had shown herself as firm as rock while the troubles of the Barclay
episode lashed around her and she had made a success of Edinburgh,

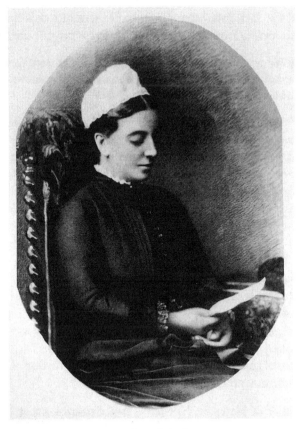

Angelique Pringle

now left in the capable hands of Frances Spencer. Unfortunately Miss Pringle's term of office was short; she was intensely religious and needed greater satisfaction than she had at that moment. Like many who found spiritual solace through the Oxford Movement, and who had been attracted to nursing through it, she now turned to the Church of Rome.

Miss Nightingale conducted a long correspondence with Mr Jowett of Balliol on the subject which is revealing as to her own metaphysical musings at this point:

> The lady we speak of I thought her much further on than I and really living up to it. But the thought that God has given me all my life has been to infuse mystic religion into forms of others... especially among women and to make them handmaidens of the Lord. Second to give them an organisation for their activity in which they could be trained. Training for women was unknown and is the discovery of the last 30 years.[33]

In spite of the fact that Miss Nightingale thought that the Church of England no longer had any meaning for most people she thought:

> some visible organisation is necessary... the question cuts very deep into me. The best and ablest woman I know is going to join the Church of Rome for no other reason.[34]

Miss Pringle did join the Church of Rome and was forced to leave St Thomas's, and so Miss Nightingale bowed to the inevitable; Miss Pringle left London to run a private nursing home in Belfast and although she continued to keep up with Miss Nightingale and her old friends, the former intimacy was over.

The next choice fell on Louise Gordon, a Nightingale nurse from Leeds, whom Miss Nightingale had not known particularly well, and nor is too clear to what extent the Fund Council was consulted. However, by the 1890s Miss Nightingale was beginning to lose interest and was more concerned with the metaphysical and less with the struggles of this world. Old friends like Benjamin Jowett, Harry Verney and her cousin Shore Smith had died and, after the age of 75, her faculties began to fail. The interest in St Thomas's was still there and she continued to send addresses to the probationers to be read by a Fund Council member, but she wrote to Miss Gordon 'Dear Matron' and, as Lytton Strachey put it,

> The author of Notes on Nursing – that classical compendium of the besetting veins of the sisterhood drawn up with detailed acrimony, the vindictive relish of a Swift – now spent long hours in composing sympathetic Addresses to probationers, whom she petted and wept over in turn.[35]

Notes

1. FN to H. Bonham Carter, BL, Add Mss 47717, 17 January, f. 147.
2. FN to H. Bonham Carter, GLRO, HI/ST/NC1.72 44b, February 1872.
3. FN to H. Bonham Carter, BL, Add Mss 47717, 17 January 1873, f. 180.
4. BL, Add Mss 47738, 16 December 1875, f. 16 (private notes).
5. Beale, L.S. in *Medical Times and Gazette*, 6 December 1873, p. 630.
6. H. Bonham Carter to FN, BL, Add Mss 47719, 4 July 1876, f. 152.
7. Croft, J., *Notes for Lectures* (Blades & Blades, London, 1874), Lecture 26, pp. 3–4.
8. FN to H. Bonham Carter, BL, Add Mss 47718, 23 March 1879, f. 9.
9. Mr Croft's Report to the Nightingale Fund Council, GLRO, HI/NTS/A2/1 (1875).
10. M. Crossland to FN, BL, Add Mss 47738, 2 June 1876, f. 42.
11. M. Crossland to FN, ibid., 27 October 1877, f. 70.

12. Nightingale, F., *Notes on Nursing* (Duckworth & Co., London, 1859), 1952 edn, p. 15.
13. FN to H. Bonham Carter, BL, Add Mss 47719, 27 January 1875, f. 84.
14. GLRO, HI/ST/C3/2.
15. GLRO, HI/ST/C37, 27 October 1877 (private notes).
16. Ibid.
17. Nuffield Provincial Hospitals Trust, *The Work of Nurses in Hospital Wards* (Nuffield Trust, London, 1953).
18. FN to H. Bonham Carter, BL, Add Mss 47719, February 1874, f. 7.
19. Royal College of Nursing, *The Problem of Providing a Continuous Nursing Service* (RCN, London, 1959).
20. M. Crossland to FN, BL, Add Mss 47738, 8 September 1877, f. 245.
21. GLRO, HI/NTS/C16 (printed leaflet), 1878.
22. FN to H. Bonham Carter, BL, Add Mss 47719, 6 July 1878, f. 245.
23. Minutes of the NFC, GLRO, A/NFC/2/1, 24 March 1879.
24. Ibid., 8 May 1883.
25. GLRO, HI/ST/NC18.26, *The Queen: The Ladies Newspaper*, Autumn 1881.
26. FN to H. Bonham Carter, BL, Add Mss 47719, 28 April 1878, f. 237.
27. FN to H. Bonham Carter, BL, Add Mss 47726, 1 May 1894, f. 6.
28. FN to H. Bonham Carter, BL, Add Mss 47721, 9 July 1887, f. 39.
29. GLRO, A/NFC/AC.75, 27 March 1885.
30. *Report of the Nightingale Fund Council*, 1886. GLRO, A/NFC/5.
31. FN to R. Williams, GLRO, HI/ST/NC3SU180, January 1873.
32. GLRO, HI/ST/NTSY27, 1. Nightingale, F., 'A Nursing Worthy' in *Hospital Nursing Supplement*.
33. FN to B. Jowett, BL, Add Mss 47785, January 1889, ff. 108–13.
34. Ibid.
35. Strachey, L., *Eminent Victorians* (Chatto & Windus, London, 1918), 1974 ed, p. 188.

11. The Fund Council and Nursing Politics

The nurses must obey the doctor's orders. Where then does the difficulty arise? It arises from this, that in matters of discipline, i.e. order and obedience, behaviour and conduct generally it is essential for the proper working of the system that nurses shall be responsible to their female superior and not the medical officer or any male officer.

H. Bonham Carter, British Medical Journal, *1879*

The original Fund Council had been selected from the Council associated with Sidney Herbert and the raising of the capital sum. The Council was large and designed to give figurative and symbolic representation and prestige. It is doubtful if Miss Nightingale saw it as a working council – otherwise she would not have expressed herself as satisfied and then go on to say:

the doctors on the Council have an absolute administrative incapacity and the three civil doctors are perfect infants in administrative matters... Dear Dawes and Colonel Jebb have both great powers but both are busy men.[1]

While Miss Nightingale was alive and active and was the controlling and executive force the administrative ability of the Council mattered little. The money was in safe hands: Lord Monteagle had been a Chancellor of the Exchequer, Edward Marjoribanks was a member of the Dudley family and a banker at Coutts, Monckton Milnes (later Lord Houghton) a Governor of the British Museum and Mr Bracebridge knew Miss Nightingale's wishes intimately and was a man of business.

The Council, as such, seldom met, and the affairs were run by a small committee, two of whom were related to both Miss Nightingale and to the secretary. It is no wonder that the journalist of *The Queen* was confused.

However, while it was policy to spend only income there was little room for manoeuvre. After the Surrey Gardens period when there were fewer probationers, the accounts over 40 years show a remarkable similarity. The income from the Trust remained much the same – about £1,500 – while the expenditure on training nurses at St Thomas's rose from £982 6s 7d in 1871 to £1,451 13s 8d but the deficit was offset by the contribution of £400 from Special Probationers in 1891, rising to £755 in 1901. The difference was that in 1871 the Fund was supplying St Thomas's with 31 probationers and in 1901 the figure had risen to 58. By now upwards of one-third of the probationers were paying for their board and lodging and giving service without a salary.

Although there is some evidence that Miss Nightingale contemplated using capital and setting up 'a School of our own' there is no suggestion in the minutes that the Council ever considered this seriously. Moreover, although the Fund Council accepted donations from time to time it apparently never considered enlarging the capital by further appeal to the public. The main reason for this seems to lie in Counsel's opinion as set out in 1874 by Mr Justice Lindley:

> And there was no special reason for retaining the Fund permanently or creating an endowment, the object had been to inaugurate a system that would be self supporting and continued by the public on account of its intrinsic merit.[2]

Both Miss Nightingale and the Council thought that the government should eventually accept the responsibility for training nurses in public hospitals, and in the voluntary system individual hospitals should set up 'normal schools'. There is plenty of evidence, both formal and informal, that the Fund Council was only too aware that it was subsidising St Thomas's hospital. More money would only increase the subsidy. The Fund Council was also aware that 'the Fund had been collected in peculiar circumstances' and it had to be cautious. Nor was it unheedful of public criticism, particularly of the way that the Fund had handed out 'douceurs to officers at St Thomas's'.[3] It would be wrong to spend more money enabling St Thomas's to do what other hospitals were now doing without a Fund.

Another reason for not enlarging the Fund was the apparent success of the paying probationer scheme. Although originally the Fund had accepted this division reluctantly, as nursing became what Miss Nightingale called 'fashionable' and more and more women were paying for other trainings like teaching, the notion of paying for a training carried intrinsic merit and kudos, an idea that nursing fostered until well into the twentieth century. It was more than the kudos of the ability to pay, it was the concept that entering the profession was so worthwhile that it was worth parental sacrifice. This was publicity in itself.

Nevertheless, both Miss Nightingale and the Council were plagued with doubts about the quality of the training and the fact that the practitioners were exploited. One answer would have been an independent school with the training of nurses divorced from the service needs of the hospital, but this is to look at history in the light of our own preoccupations. In 1860 the state of medicine did not warrant an academic training for nurses and Miss Nightingale herself was adamant, and rightly so, that nursing should be taught on the wards and on the district. The School of Nursing had to be attached to a hospital and, in spite of *The Lancet*'s comments, would any hospital drive a less hard bargain? The Fund Council agonised over the problem for years, but did not solve it and it remains largely unsolved.

The Council, which only met as such in 1861 and 1863, became depleted by deaths. Sir Joshua Jebb had died suddenly in 1863, Lord Monteagle, a trustee, in 1864, the Dean of Hereford and Sir John Liddell died four years later and Mr Bracebridge followed in 1871. It seems that from 1872 Edward Marjoribanks, a valued trustee, was incapacitated from attending. Lord Houghton wrote:

> the transference of stock brought strongly before me the peculiar and inconvenient condition of your Trust. Two of the four Trustees, Lord Monteagle and Bracebridge, are dead. Poor Marjoribanks is dying bankrupt and my life is by no means a good one. I think you should consider with H.B.C. the advisability of constituting a new Trust, if you wish that condition of things to continue.[4]

At the same time Lord Houghton wrote to Henry Bonham Carter saying that he would work with any person Miss Nightingale might select.[5]

This led to the appointment by Miss Nightingale of three new trustees: the Duke of Westminster, the Earl of Pembroke and William Rathbone MP. The Council, which was now synonymous with the Committee, had dwindled to the Chairman, Sir Harry Verney, Sir John Forbes Clark, Sir John McNeill, William Bowman and William Spottiswoode.[6] All were busy men and it is not surprising that with so small a committee the meetings were at times inquorate. Curiously enough this does not seem to have disturbed Miss Nightingale's administrative mind. However, to overcome this in 1879 Sir William Wyatt, the Poor Law reformer from St Pancras, joined the Council together with Sir William Muir and Mr Rathbone. In 1889, after the

Council had again been reduced by four deaths, Edmund Boulnois MP and the Reverend Dacre Craven were added, both of whom were connected with the Poor Law and Dacre Craven also with District Nursing. The aim now seemed to be to have a Council which represented the different interests of the Fund.

In spite of her emphasis on the need for women's education and her association with Jowett Miss Nightingale did not, apparently, see fit to appoint an educationalist to the Council nor yet a woman. The Metropolitan Asylums Board were appointing women to their Boards and Dr Ayers thinks this was due to Miss Nightingale's influence,[7] and there were possibilities within her own circle. Barbara Leigh Smith (later Barbara Bodichon), who was involved with the educational side of the women's movement and Bedford College, was a Nightingale cousin; Ann Clough, the head of Newnham in 1875, was the sister of the beloved Arthur; and Miss Nightingale was a friend of Dr Elizabeth Blackwell and her circle.[8] There is something a little illogical about the insistence of putting 'all power (in nursing matters) into the hand of one female head' and yet excluding women from the governing body.

The answer seems to be that Miss Nightingale did not see nursing as a mainly educational process but rather a moral and character training. Although originally a staunch supporter of women's property rights as she grew older she lost patience with the women's movement and many associated with it. In July 1867 John Stuart Mill, whom she admired and corresponded with, asked her to become a member of the Committee of the London National Society for Women's Suffrage but, although her name would have meant so much, she refused:

> That women should have suffrage I think no one can be more convinced than I... but it will be years before you obtain suffrage. And in the meantime there are evils which press more hardly on women than the want of suffrage. Till a married woman can have possession of her own property there can be no justice.[9]

Miss Nightingale was irritated by the clamour for votes because she thought that the main problem for women was to provide them with training for worthwhile work, and the most worthwhile work in Miss Nightingale's eyes was, of course, nursing. This was 'womanly work' and did not challenge men. Like Octavia Hill, who wrote that 'political power would militate against women's usefulness in the large field of public work',[10] Miss Nightingale was exasperated by the desire to emulate men while there was women's work to be done. However towards the end of her life she relented and in 1877 she actually signed a petition urging the admission of women to medical degrees at the University of London. Later, while admitting to being 'enraged by vociferous ladies talking on things they know nothing at all about', she confessed that she had not given enough thought to the rank and file of women who had none of her advantages. Although the Fund Council were men, most were liberals and some (like Lord Houghton) supported the feminist cause. It is noticeable that the Council used Emily Faithfull's Victoria Printing Press, which was founded in 1876 as a Women's Printing Society, to provide work for women.

The short answer to the absence of women on the governing body was that Miss Nightingale preferred working with men. The diatribe on 'widow's caps' – 'women crave for being loved, not loving – they scream at you all day long, they are incapable of giving any in return for they cannot remember your affairs long enough to do so',[11] gives some idea of Miss Nightingale's opinion of her own sex. It is significant that throughout her life Miss Nightingale's favourite women, including relatives like Aunt Mai, all sooner or later fell from favour unlike the men favourites who seldom did so. The other reason for choosing men was probably blatantly political; she wanted a Council with influence in high places, which was something women did not have.

As early as 1866 Henry Bonham Carter had suggested to the Council that they should be presented on the Court of Governors of St Thomas's Hospital. William Spottiswoode had been nominated and had agreed but nothing was done.[12] Although there is nothing in the Fund Council minutes, in 1872 there appears in the records of St Thomas's the fact that 'On December 19th 1872 Sir H. Verney, Sir J.F. Clark, Wm. Bowman esq., Wm. Spottiswoode esq., and H. Bonham Carter esq. who have presented £250 to the hospital are elected governors.'[13]

Later Henry Bonham Carter became a member of the Grand Council, served on the Almoner's Committee and was clearly considered an expert on nursing matters. How far this helped the working arrangements between the Fund and the officials of the hospital is not clear, but during the later years of the century the relationship seems better. Probably the Fund Council had made its point, and it was now a fact that the Nightingale School did bring kudos and advantage to the hospital. All the arrangements for the School were made through the treasurer who controlled the purse-strings and at one stage the Fund Council seriously considered canvassing its own nominee as treasurer but nothing came of this proposal.

In its report of 1886 the Fund Council made a great point of the missionary effect of the Nightingale School but by then there was competition. There were older 'trainings' like King's College and Charing Cross hospitals with their origins in sisterhoods; there were those like the Westminster where a Lady Superintendent acted as an agent and supplied a staff of nurses for a fixed fee, and there were schools like the Middlesex, and later the London and Guy's hospitals, where reforming matrons had evolved their own schemes and, because they had no Fund, tended to have more paying probationers. By now trainees from these hospitals were applying for, and getting, superintendent's posts. For example Miss Lückes from the Middlesex and Westminster to the London, Miss Thorold from University College to the Middlesex, Miss Manson (later Mrs Bedford Fenwick) from the London to St Bartholomew's and Miss Burt from St John's to Guy's Hospital. These in their turn set up reformed trainings with variations on the Nightingale theme.

One effect of hospitals taking more Lady Probationers was the demand for a more scientific training. Twenty-five years had seen many changes since the Medical Registration Act of 1858, other professions (accountants and architects, for example) were seeking charters and the teaching profession was pressing for registration to 'protect the public'. In 1864 a School's Enquiry Commission had been set up and thanks to the strenuous efforts, and the evidence of women like Emily Davies, Miss Buss and Miss Beale this led to an improvement in the endowment system and the opening in towns all over the country of good inexpensive schools – high schools modelled on Miss Buss's schools – and to the establishment of institutions of higher education for women.[14] By the 1880s some of the intake into nursing were the products of such schools. Eva Lückes, for example, had been to Cheltenham College and more and more of these women would look for equal opportunities with men. However there was no central organisation to co-ordinate the views of nurses other than, of course, the Fund Council. But Miss Nightingale's training was primarily aimed at making an intelligent working-class girl into a practical nurse who was not much concerned with parity with the medical profession. Moreover many of the early Lady Probationers, wherever they were educated, were inspired by religious and spiritual motives and not concerned with status. Therefore there were many shades of opinion as to the right attributes for nursing and the path that the nursing profession should take.

The new reformers who wanted nursing to be more 'scientific' pressed for a longer and more rigorous training. Miss Nightingale was against this because she thought, with her experience of St Thomas's, that a longer training would mean longer exploitation by the hospital. If the Fund Council could not stop this what hope had hospitals without a fund? Nevertheless the reformers had a point; every hospital of any size was trumpeting a nurse training scheme, some offered a systematic course with lectures, but many were 'earning and learning schemes' with more emphasis on earning than learning. Some order was needed and the new reformers now pressed the idea of state registration for trained nurses.

Setting up nurse training schemes had involved wresting some power from the doctors because the probationers were 'under the control of one female head' and nurses were moved from ward to ward for experience, a practice to which the doctors often objected. There were disputes with the doctors which led reformers like Mrs Bedford Fenwick, who were also ardent suffragettes, to say, 'The nurse question is the woman question' and at this point nursing touched the women's movement. In the conflict not all the new-style nurses used their independence tactfully and the Lonsdale Affair at Guy's Hospital reverberated far and wide.

Early in 1880, Miss Lonsdale, a trained lady nurse under the reforming zeal of Margaret Burt, the Matron, wrote an article in the *Nineteenth Century Journal* in which she described the old-style nurse as ignorant and immoral, and went on to accuse the honorary doctors at Guy's as opposing the change because of

> their anxiety lest their malpractice should be exposed by women of refinement and culture. Are not practices indulged in by medical men and permitted by them to the members of the medical school, which it is understood had better not be named beyond the wards of the hospital? If talked of by old nurses no one took any notice. But the pressure of refined, intelligent women in the wards imposes a kind of moral restraint.[15]

This unfortunate article was taken up by correspondence in the *British Medical Journal* and dismissed as ridiculous, a writer claiming that

> Lady nurses do not make first rate nurses, they are essentially amateurish... ladies take to nursing, as a rule, from some slightly morbid motive, they are disappointed or they want something to kill the ennui or they have religious convictions.

The writer sums up what he and many of his colleagues would have seen as the heart of the matter, that any system should provide a staff of thoroughly trained nurses

> to carry out the order of the doctor, to whom they should look, *and to whom they alone should look,* for orders and guidance... there is no reason why there should not be a superintendent who would report to the medical man any dereliction of duty she may detect in any nurse under his special charge.[16]

The Nightingale message does not seem to have reached Manchester from whence this letter came.

The correspondence stirred up a hornet's nest and a great deal of emotional irrelevance which indicated the professional insecurity of both doctors and nurses. After 20 years the principles enunciated by the Fund Council were by no means fully accepted. In May Miss Pringle replied with a reasoned article in the *Edinburgh Medical Journal* which was supported by the surgeon Mr Joseph Bell, and may be said to represent the Fund's line. Miss Pringle's point was that in the past conditions for nurses had been so bad that it was no wonder that they fell asleep or were unable to do their work, and indeed, in spite of the appalling conditions the old-style nurses were 'often clever, dutiful, cheerful and kind, endowed above all with that motherliness of nature which is the most precious attribute of a nurse'. Miss Pringle then set out what was needed for those attributes to flourish, but she wisely concluded that good conditions of themselves did not make for good nursing and that 'it will ever be an uphill task to provide good and devoted nurses in sufficient numbers'. Turning to Miss Lonsdale's complaint she said, with some sagacity, 'my experience with doctors has been different and nurses often experienced the kind of behaviour they themselves attracted or merited'. Mr Bell, riding in like Don Quixote, pointed out to his colleagues that probationers had to be moved for the sake of their training, but at Edinburgh

> The medical staff wish to help the lady superintendent to train her nurses and the lady superintendent sees that the real object of the nursing staff is to help the physicians and surgeons to care for the sick poor; not to wear any particular raiment, however becoming: not even to pin up coverlids in any particular way, however inscrutable; not to talk of a vocation but to live one.[17]

Such words of wisdom should have quelled the controversy, but unfortunately in many places it smouldered on and was the undercurrent of the registration debate with which the Fund Council was soon to be involved.

The problem of recognising who was a trained nurse was taken up by Henry Burdett of the Hospitals' Association and in 1887 a meeting was called to discuss the formation of a Nursing Section of the Association. The meeting, according to Abel-Smith, was stormy and it ended with Mrs Bedford Fenwick, lately matron of St Bartholomew's, inviting the disaffected ladies to her house in Manchester Square where the British Nurses' Association was born.[18] Meanwhile the group that remained with the Hospitals' Association set about establishing a Directory for Nurses which was open to those who had worked for a year in a hospital or infirmary, who had been trained in the duties of a nurse and who had a testimonial of good character. The members of the Registration Committee included Mrs Wardroper, Miss

Vincent and Miss Lückes, the young matron from the London who was now in communication with Miss Nightingale, and which seems to indicate that, in spite of her abuse of Mr Burdett, Miss Nightingale was not originally against such a Directory. The Directory was boycotted by the British Nurses' Association but it remains a valuable source for researchers.

The British Nurses' Association was set up with an elaborate constitution and a General Council consisting mainly of London matrons and doctors with the aim of state registration for nurses after a three-year training. To this end it set up its own register of nurses who produced evidence of a year's training before 1889, and satisfactory professional attainment and personal character. This allowed, as members, those Lady Probationers who at that time had done only a year's training. After 1889 the criterion was a three-year training and this excluded the Fund's nurses.

In 1890, in response to a petition from the Charity Organisation Society, a Select Committee of the House of Lords was set up to enquire into the work of the Metropolitan Hospitals.[19] A large proportion of the evidence centred on a dispute at the London Hospital where it was said that first-year probationers were given too much responsibility and were left in charge, and that they were overworked and underfed. Miss Nightingale and her cousin, General Nicholson, who was a Governor of the London Hospital, supported Miss Lückes, but much of the controversy turned on the attacks made by Mrs Bedford Fenwick in the *Nursing Record*, the paper she edited, on the one-year training, and therefore on the Fund Council.[20]

Mr Rathbone, on behalf of the Fund, gave evidence on the lines indicated by Miss Nightingale. This seems to have been sufficient for the Committee to find against registration. The Lords eventually reported in 1892 and although in general they found the London hospitals well administered and supported the authority of the matron in nursing matters, they recommended that nurse training should be extended to three years. They also suggested that no nurse should work more than an eight-hour day, something that did not happen for another 60 years. All hospitals were advised to follow the example of the London and Guy's and join the National Pension Fund for Nurses, that one innovation by Mr Burdett that Miss Nightingale admired.

The British Nurses' Association's position was now strengthened by the fact that Princess Christian Helena, the third daughter of Queen Victoria, had consented to be their patron. 'This', as Mr Rathbone said, 'made things awkward for the anti-registrationists.' The Association, without much regard for the logistics of need, wanted to confine nursing to the 'educated classes', to test a three-year training by external examination and to charge five guineas as a registration fee, a sum equivalent to a quarter of the first-year salary for a trained nurse. Miss Nightingale considered these requirements unrealistic:

> Nursing has to nurse living bodies and spirits. It cannot be formulated like engineering. It cannot be numbered and registered like arithmetic or population. It cannot be tested by public examination, though it may be tested by current supervision.[21]

In her large correspondence with Jowett on the subject she complains that after 30 years, which she reckoned to be the lifetime of modern nursing, a 'buying and selling spirit had entered' and in a paper to a Congress of Women's Work held at Chicago in 1895 she wrote about the dangers to which nursing was subject. It was 'a profession rather than a calling... Fashion on one side, and a consequent want of earnestness; mere money getting on the other side, and a mechanical view of nursing.'[22] It is interesting that Miss Nightingale is now using the word 'profession' as pejorative. Paradoxically she saw the registrationists as wanting to lower the standard, whereas they saw themselves as wanting to raise it and make nursing more exclusive. However, Miss Nightingale's main fear was that the patient work of years would be undone and nursing would be divided against itself – 'I have terror lest the B.N.A.'s and the anti-B.N.A.'s should form hostile camps'[23] – and she goes on to compare the bitterness that was then being generated by the Home Rule Bill. The amount of correspondence on the subject shows the extent to which Miss Nightingale worried about it. She was all too well aware of the shortcomings of the present system but these could not be rectified by making the training three years and by testing by some outside examination. 'What has been meant by a three year training has been asked in vain', she wrote to her cousin.[24]

Nevertheless if there had to be two camps Miss Nightingale took every precaution to ensure that hers was the stronger. The British Nurses' Association prepared a preliminary register which Miss Nightingale analysed and compared with hospital registers and found discrepancies; names were included on the BNA register that were not acknowledged by the training schools. Now, having failed to get support for an Act of Parliament to make registration compulsory, the Association appealed to Sir Michael Hicks-Beach at the Board of Trade for the Association to be a public company and the memorandum and articles included the aim of setting up a register of trained nurses. Coached by Miss Nightingale, Sir Harry Verney saw Sir Michael and presented a statement against the articles and the

Board of Trade duly refused the request of the BNA. Miss Nightingale then wrote to Mr Rathbone informing him that the licence had been refused and to enquire whether this was done

> because it was not within his [Sir Michael's] competence or because he had decided on the merits of the case. If the later then you should ensure that Sir Michael was consulted if the B.N.A. apply for a Royal Charter.[25]

Then, with merited faith in the delaying powers of a Royal Commission, she suggested that this might well be the best way for the government to get out of the difficulty. Miss Nightingale rightly divined the next step; the Association asked for, and were granted, permission to use the title Royal, then they played their trump card and got their royal patron to petition for a Royal Charter.

The petition was referred to a Select Committee of the Privy Council in 1892 and heard by two judges and two Law Lords. Two outstanding petitions were presented against the Charter, the first from the Nightingale Fund Council and the second from 'Executive Officers, Matrons, Lady Superintendents and Principal Assistants of the London and Provincial Hospitals and Nurse Training Schools and Members of the Medical Profession'; the list of signatures which occupies three pages was headed by Florence Nightingale's.

The petition prepared by the Fund Council runs into 87 pages and was signed by Henry Bonham Carter, Eva Lückes and Emmeline Stains, now the Lady Superintendent of the Nurses' Training School, Liverpool.[26] Other training schools to petition against the Charter were the Westminster, King's College Hospital, St Mary's Paddington, Charing Cross, the Seaman's Hospital at Greenwich, St Marylebone, St Pancras at Highgate, the Royal Free, Edinburgh Royal Infirmary, Bristol Royal Infirmary, Dublin Infirmary, Leeds Infirmary, the Manchester Royal Infirmary, the Metropolitan and National Nursing Association and certain members of St Bartholomew's, indicating that Mrs Bedford Fenwick's ideas were not universally acceptable in the hospital where she had been matron.

The Fund Council's case is important because it sets out succinctly the Fund's philosophy towards nursing and, unlike the Association, it emphasises the difference between nursing and medicine. The achievements of the Fund are set out by recapitulating much of the 1886 report. It was stressed that the aim of the Fund had been to raise the character of nurses, to cultivate and protect their moral qualities, and then to promote such means of practical and scientific training as might enable them intelligently to obey the orders of medical men.

The means of achieving this aim had been the supplying of a Nurses' Home where good women could live and enjoy good accommodation, better food and shorter hours under the supervision of educated matrons, and the selection of probationers with good health and the qualities of gentleness, tact, presence of mind and other qualities without which no training can succeed. To all this had to be added a methodical system of practical and technical training in the wards by head nurses and especially appointed medical staff. The training had to be not less than one year with a further period of two or three years under direction. During the training there had to be continual assessment of the character and efficiency of the probationers kept in a complete and confidential record. Each training school needed to keep in touch with its trainees and should be able to provide a complete register. Mr Bonham Carter admitted that not all these aims had been obtained by the Fund but they remained the desideratum.

The petition went on to point out that there was no concurrence of opinion as to what constituted an adequate training or what the minimum qualification should be, and much longer experience was needed before a register could be contemplated; indeed, the Hospitals' Association had looked at the possibility of such a register and had reported adversely.

The petition concluded by setting out the reasons against the Charter. First, a register was not adapted to the calling of nurses for the sick and nursing was not analogous with medicine. Second, if there was to be a register then there must be statutory power, for power under the authority of a Charter would be mischievous, for the Royal British Nurses' Association would have real, if indirect, power of controlling the education of the whole nursing profession. Moreover, it was asserted, the Association was by no means representative and furthermore it had not the means of discharging the duties a Charter would place upon it. In effect the petition was saying *Quis custodiet ipsos custodes?*

Part of the submission was based on the booklet *Is a General Register for Nurses Desirable?* by Henry Bonham Carter[27] and a paper prepared by Mr Rathbone and Miss Lückes. In this paper he argued that nursing should not be compared with medicine. All that medical registration had told the public was that there had been an absence of bad conduct and that the doctor had passed certain examinations. Had registration, of itself, he asked, done anything to raise the status of the profession? But nursing, he stressed, could not be examined like medical knowledge, it was essentially practical and technical, and above all nursing depended on moral qualities and attributes like patience and kindness that cannot be tested. The status of nursing had risen not because nurses had become cleverer but because they were

more moral and worthy people, and in this respect nursing was difference from medicine, or indeed from midwifery; it was wider and
depended far more on the intangible attributes.

The Fund's case was presented by Sir Richard Webster, and Miss
Nightingale sent a blow-by-blow account to Sir Harry Verney. At first
it was feared that the Select Committee would favour the petition for a
Charter especially as the Lords had already accepted the idea of a three-
year training. But although the Royal British Nurses' Association were
eventually jubilant because they were granted a Charter, it was a hollow
victory because it did nothing to give them the right to maintain a register. Instead the words 'the maintenance of a list of persons who may
have applied to have their names entered there as nurses' were substi-
tuted. This is not quite what the Association wanted.

When the smoke cleared it was obvious that little had changed and
the Association had to take up cudgels again in an endeavour to get
Parliamentary time for a Registration Bill – a fight that was to last
nearly another 30 years. Once the petition against the Charter was
paid for, and Miss Nightingale made a considerable personal contribution, the Fund set about mending some fences. Miss Nightingale
continued to work behind the scenes schooling her medical friends and
sometimes placating her enemies. Soon there was a serious and acri-
monious rift in the ranks of the Royal British Nurses' Association and
the Bedford Fenwicks left in high dudgeon. This made it easier to
make overtures to Princess Christian who in 1894 produced a scheme
for enrolling a Voluntary Nurses Corps for War through the hospitals
and had written to Miss Nightingale for advice. 'This', wrote Miss
Nightingale, was an opportunity for 'A flag of peace to the princess
and getting away from all this bickering and lying that does so much
harm to the cause.'[28]

It was not only the Fund Council that was at the centre of dissension. Mrs Bedford Fenwick now set about starting other organisations
to further her objectives, and these new organisations clashed not only
with the Royal British Nurses' Association, at least for the time being,
but also with Mr Burdett and the Hospitals' Association. Both
Mrs Bedford Fenwick and Mr Burdett were implacable enemies and
gave no quarter attacking one another in a near libellous manner in
their respective journals.[29] But from now on, except for the occasional
anti-registrationist shot, the Fund Council kept itself out of the fray of
nursing politics. The Nightingale system went on as before.

Assets on the 25th December, 1881, £48,000 New Three per Cents.; £1300 Consols; £1900 Great Northern Railway Debenture Stock; Cash on Deposit and Current Account at Bankers, less Bills due, £1350 2s. 4d.

INCOME AND EXPENDITURE OF THE NIGHTINGALE FUND FOR THE YEAR ENDING 25TH DECEMBER, 1901.

RECEIPTS	£	s.	d.
Balance from last Account (including advance payments from Probationers)	239	5	8
Income from Trust Funds	1,490	16	5
Donation	10	10	0
Payments by Special Probationers	755	0	0
	£2,495	12	1

EXPENDITURE	£	s.	d.
Expenses of training Hospital Nurses at St. Thomas' Hospital	1,451	13	8
Probationers' Uniform	75	17	1
Contribution to Expenses of Training School at St. Marylebone Infirmary	198	5	0
Gratuities to Certified Nurses	248	0	0
Pension	50	0	0
Grant to Metropolitan Nursing Association for District Training	100	0	0
Advertisements, Printing, Stationery, Books, Clerical Work, Secretary's Salary, and Petty Cash	114	1	0
Balance carried forward (including advance payments from Probationers)	257	15	4
	£2,495	12	1

Assets on the 25th December, 1901, £56,424 4s. London Country 2¹/₂ per Cent. Stock. £2,533 6s. 8d. Great Northern Railway Three Per Cent. Debenture Stock. Cash at Bankers £832 5s. 4d., less Bills due, £574 10s. 0d., leaving a net balance of £257 15s. 4d.

Examined with vouchers and found correct by COOPER BROTHERS & Co., *Chartered Accountants, 8th May, 1903.*

Examples from the accounts of the Nightingale Fund

ABSTRACT OF ACCOUNTS FOR YEAR ENDING
DEC 24, 1863.

DR.	£	s.	d.	CR.	£	s.	d.
Balance, June 24 1863	1,226	17	7	Expenses of Training			
Income from Trust				Hospital Nurses at			
Funds, viz., £200 South				St. Thomas's Hospital	518	10	5
Australian Bonds,				Expenses of Training			
£48,000 New Three per				Midwifery Nurses for			
Cents., £1,000 Consols	1,426	8	6	the Poor at King's			
				College Hospital	420	0	0
				Advertisements, Print-			
				ing, &c	41	17	0
				Secretary	50	0	0
				Balance	1,622	18	8
	£2, 653	6	1		£2,653		1

(NB. 1863 is the first year accounts show the income)

ABSTRACT OF ACCOUNTS FOR THE YEAR ENDING
25TH DECEMBER, 1881.

RECEIPTS	£	s.	d.
Balance from last Account	1272	6	9
Income From Trust Funds	1576	11	3
Payments by Special Probationers	329	12	0
	£3178	10	0

EXPENDITURE	£	s.	d.
Expenses of training Hospital Nurses at St. Thomas' Hospital	1396	18	6
Clothing of Probationers	73	11	11
Gratuities to Certified Nurses	122	0	0
Contribution to District Nursing Associations	50	0	0
Advertisements, Printing, Books, Secretary's and Clerk's Salary, and Petty Cash	185	17	3
Balance	1350	2	4
	£3178	10	0

Notes

1. FN to Sidney Herbert, *Herbert Papers*, Wilton House, 26 May 1859.
2. Minutes of the Council. The Opinion of Mr Justice Lindley, GLRO/A/NFC/2/1, 5 August 1874.
3. *Pall Mall Magazine*, February 1866; *The Lancet*, 31 March 1866; see also *The Queen Magazine*, Autumn 1881.
4. Lord Houghton 'Dear Friend'(?) to Sir H. Verney, GLRO, A/NFC/7/2, 18 November 1878.
5. Lord Houghton to H. Bonham Carter, GLRO, HI/ST/NC, 18.12 (53), November 1878.
6. *Report of the Nightingale Fund Council* (year ending 25 December 1877).
7. Ayers, G., *England's First State Hospital* (Wellcome Institute, London, 1971), p. 132.
8. Kamm, J., *Rapiers and Battleaxes – The Women's Movement and its Aftermath* (George Allen & Unwin, London, 1966), Chapter 3.
9. Huxley, E., *Florence Nightingale* (Wiedenfeld & Nicholson, London, 1975), p. 220, quoting FN to J.S. Mill, 11 August 1867.
10. Kamm, *Rapiers and Battleaxes*, p. 128.
11. Cook, Sir E., *The Life of Florence Nightingale* (Macmillan, London, 1913), vol. 2, p. 15, quoting FN's letter to Madame Mohl, 13 December 1861.
12. Wm. Spottiswoode to H. Bonham Carter, GLRO, HI/ST/NC18.6(42), January 1866.
13. Records of St Thomas's Hospital, GLRO, HI/ST/A6/16.
14. Kamm, *Rapiers and Battleaxes*, p. 57–9.
15. Cameron, H.C., *Mr Guy's Hospital* (Longmans, Green & Co., London, 1954), p. 205.
16. *British Medical Journal*, 17 March 1880, GLRO, HI/ST/NC15/6.
17. Report from the *Edinburgh Medical Journal*, 'Nurses and Doctors', May 1880, GLRO, HI/ST/NC18.1(6).
18. Abel-Smith, B., *A History of the Nursing Profession* (Heinemann, London, 1960), p. 68ff.
19. *Third Report from the Select Committee on Metropolitan Hospitals* (1892).
20. Clark-Kennedy, A.E., *The London*, vol. 2 (Pitman Medical Press, London, 1962), p. 105–26. See also *The Nursing Record* (Editorials), 1890.
21. Rathbone, W., *A History of District Nursing*, with an introduction by F. Nightingale from which this quote is taken (Macmillan & Co., London, 1890).
22. Cook, *Florence Nightingale*, p. 365.
23. Woodham-Smith, C., *Florence Nightingale* (Constable, London, 1860), p. 570 quoting the correspondence with Jowett.
24. FN to H. Bonham Carter, GLRO, HI/ST/NC1/89, 20 April 1889.
25. FN to Wm. Rathbone, GLRO/ HI/ST/NC1/91.3, 25 May 1891.

26. *The Case for the Opposition to the Royal British Nurses' Association*, GLRO, HI/ST/NTS/A17.1, November 1892.
27. GLRO, A/NFC/21/1, July 1888.
28. FN to H. Bonham Carter, BL, Add Mss 47726, 2 May 1894, f. 9.
29. Abel-Smith, B., *A History of the Nursing Profession* (Heinemann, London, 1960), p. 68f.

12. The Nightingale Legacy at the Beginning of the Twentieth Century

It may well be said that the seed sown by Miss Nightingale through the means of the Fund has been mainly instrumental in raising the calling of nurses to the position it now holds.

> *Report of the Nightingale Fund Council, 1910.*
> *(On the death of Miss Nightingale.)*

Although the change probably occurred slowly there is evidence that towards the end of the nineteenth century the increased demand for nursing service altered the position of probationers to their contract with the Fund Council. As antisepsis and asepsis became widely used and accepted hospitals could offer new therapies and safer care. With the knowledge of the germ theory patient care improved and principles of isolation helped to confine the infection that once swept though the wards. There was a shift from home care to hospitals which now attracted a growing middle-class clientele. Hospitals, originally intended for the poor sick, now had private patients' wards and wings. As more nursing schools opened all over the country, hospital administrators wooed fee-paying patients by replacing attendants with respectable student nurses:

> The reforms that Nightingale and others had instituted earlier had produced a worker that neatly suited these requirements. Indeed some historians have suggested that earlier hospital reform in itself had accelerated the use of the hospital. Observing the new order that trained nurses brought to hospital wards doctors may have brought middle class patients to hospitals more readily.[1]

St Thomas's Hospital was not an exception to this change; in fact it had been in the forefront of the controversy in the debate concerning remuneration for doctors for paying patients and the extent to which this was depriving general practitioners of their living.

Nevertheless, in March 1881 the St Thomas's Home for Paying Patients opened its doors.[2] This was a further incentive to the governors to press for more middle-class, educated probationers.

By 1890 Miss Gordon, the matron, was admitting up to 50 probationers a year of whom a third were now Specials.[3] This entailed the Fund in extra financial outlay for salaries and board and lodging and in 1891 Mr Bonham Carter wrote to the treasurer, 'There is no question, but that payment for probationers must be largely diminished... last year showed an excess of expenditure over income of £509 13s 9d... '[4] A conference must have taken place between the Fund and the hospital authorities because in March 1892 Mr Bonham Carter wrote that he would pay the account on the 'basis of the September proposals' which were

> That the Nightingale Fund shall (1) pay for the whole items of the expense of instruction and also the salaries of the probationers, in fact all the items in the account except the board of the probationers, but including the board of Miss Crossland and her assistant. (2) Shall credit the hospital with all payments made by paying probationers, and it shall be left to further consideration what further sums the Fund shall pay towards the balance of free probationers.[5]

This, then is the principle of the 1891 agreement. The Fund gave the hospital the money it received from paying probationers in exchange for the hospital taking responsibility for all board and lodging expenses except those of the Home sister. On the calculation of about 20 ordinary probationers and 13 paying Specials the deal was finely balanced. This 1891 agreement is important because, except for minor modifications, it remained the basis of the agreement between the Fund and St Thomas's until 1937. From 1891 it was the hospital authorities that had the interest in the number of paying probationers, an interest they now had in common with other London teaching hospitals.

Apart from the change in the Fund's commitment for financing the probationers a change in the contract to give service had occurred because in 1904 Mr Bonham Carter wrote to the treasurer about the need to amend the regulations for probationers:

> I have had to recast the regulations for the admission of probationers ... The existing regulations have for many years not been consistent with the practice that has grown up in regards to passing on the whole of the probationers to the hospital staff first as 'extra' nurses, then as staff nurses. The clause remained that at the close of a year's training they would be required to enter into service in a hospital or infirmary or such a situation as may be offered them... they naturally ask whether they are liable to be sent away...[6]

From this it is clear that as early as the 1890s all the service stipulated in clause 6 of the contract was now given at St Thomas's. Although Miss Nightingale and the Fund Council adhered to the principle of a one-year training the first step towards a three-year training in the same hospital had been taken.

By the beginning of the twentieth century the need for nursing staff had again increased and more probationers were taken on by the matron. To meet the increased cost the Fund made economies; candidates admitted after 1900 ceased to be given gratuities and, after much heart searching, a certificate was given instead – a course against which Mr Bonham Carter had set his face for years because, as he pointed out in the registration debate, a certificate was only valid on the day it was issued. Two years later the Fund ceased to supply uniform dresses for paying probationers,[7] but this was not enough and in 1903 it was resolved that 'A letter be sent to the treasurer concerning the increased number of probationers whose salaries were paid by the Nightingale Fund requesting that a limit be agreed.'[8] Presumably some bargaining took place because the Committee had sought 20 as the limit but in the end it was agreed that 'The sum to be paid by the Nightingale Fund to St Thomas's Hospital for salaries was to be restricted to twenty four probationers, the hospital paying the excess.'[9]

The ever increasing demand for probationers and rising costs, especially those relating to the maintenance of probationers, were gradually limiting the proportion of the training costs that the Fund could afford to pay out of its income. On the other hand, as Henry Bonham Carter was soon to argue, there was a query as to what were 'training costs'; the three-year contract of service was now supplying St Thomas's, and other similar schools, with much of its nursing service. Moreover it can be seen from the timetable that the young probationers were on the wards for ten hours a day, longer hours than those permitted by the Factory Act.

Although diaries had ceased and we no longer have the hour-by-hour occupation of the probationers, as late as 1918 there is a notice to probationers signed by Miss Lloyd-Still instructing them how to apply for cleaning materials which include 'Soap, Brass Polish, Locker Polish, etc.'.[10] From this it can be fairly assumed that the probationers now did much of the cleaning. Miss Nightingale was no longer around to thunder 'this is hospital work, not training'. Interestingly enough the list of duties drawn up by Mrs Wardroper and Mr Bonham Carter in 1879 does not include cleaning duties other than 'cleaning urinals and bedpans'[11] and the diaries do not indicate that the probationers polished brass. The evidence suggests that by the beginning of the twentieth century, as the number of probationers increased and ward

Alterations asked for by Miss Gordon and Miss Crossland 21/2/91
St Thomas's Hospital Timetable for the Probationers in the 'Nightingale Home'

For Those on Day Duty

Rise	Breakfast	Wards	Dinner	Wards	Exercise	Tea	Wards	Home	Supper	Bed
6 a.m.	6½ a.m.	7 a.m.	¼ to 1 p.m.	1.30 p.m.	10½ a.m. to a ¼ to 1 p.m. or 3 to 5 p.m.	5 p.m.	6 p.m.	8½ p.m.	9 p.m.	10 p.m.

For Those on (Special) Night Duty, according to Time of Year

Rise	Tea	Wards	Breakfast	Wards	Home	Exercise	Dinner	Bed
9 p.m. or 5 p.m.	9½ p.m. or 9 p.m.	10 p.m. to 7 a.m.	7 a.m.	8 a.m.	10 a.m.	11 a.m. to ¼ to 1 p.m. 6¼ to 8 p.m.	¼ to 5½ p.m. 1 p.m. or 10 a.m. to 5 p.m.	2 to 9 p.m. or

1891

Probationers will be released from Ward Duties (unless in attendance on special cases) for an interval of 1½ or 2 hours on two days in the Week, for the purpose of class instruction.

Courses of Lectures suitable for Nurses are given by the Medical Instructor, and also by two of the Hospital Professors, on Medicine, Anatomy, Physiology and Chemistry.

During the Week, Prayers are read in the Wards at 8 a.m., and in the Nightingale Home at ¼ before 9 p.m.

On Sunday the Probationers are expected to attend Divine Service in the Hospital Chapel at 10.30 a.m.

Note: Compare this with the timetable for 1862 on page 48. Little has changed, and almost the same timetable was in use in the 1920s.

maids became more expensive, so the probationers took on more cleaning tasks.

In 1904 the Fund Council gave up its last commitment to a training scheme outside St Thomas's Hospital: 'The Secretary of the Nightingale Fund informed the Board of St Marylebone that it would only pay gratuities as per existing arrangements for probationers trained at St Marylebone and that payments by the Fund will cease...'[12] Arrangements were made for the Metropolitan Common Poor Law Fund to take over the payments for training. The official reason for ending the contract was that the probationers trained at St Marylebone did not, in many cases, do what was intended and further the cause of Poor Law nursing; instead they went into private nursing. This tendency was not, however, confined to St Marylebone but reflected the new demand for, and the outlet for, trained nurses. The most likely reason for withdrawal was one of economy, and that Henry Bonham Carter, who had long advocated that the government should be responsible for training nurses in public hospitals, decided that after the Poor Law Order of 1897 the time for this had now arrived at Marylebone.

Because Miss Nightingale insisted that nurse training should be practical and strictly ward based, she disapproved of the idea of a 'Preliminary Training School'. She was particularly acerbic about the one started by Mrs Strong at the Glasgow Royal Hospital in 1893 where she said the pupils 'lacked the moral training of the Home'. Two years later when her friend, Eva Lückes, proposed such a scheme she wrote:

> I am most anxious to hear what you propose with regard to the teaching of probationers anatomy, physiology etc. before they enter the wards for practical training. It is a system I have always dreaded. But no doubt you will convince me.[13]

Miss Lückes did not convince her and there was no Preliminary School at St Thomas's until the year of Miss Nightingale's death. The change when it did come seems to have been prompted, not by the Fund Council, but by Mr Wainwright, the hospital treasurer, for among Mr Bonham Carter's papers there is a significant memorandum which reads:

> Notwithstanding the care taken in selecting candidates, it is increasingly realised that sufficient means are not afforded by the present practice of testing the suitability of candidates. The result has been a very large number of failures and withdrawals have occurred amongst probationers during their first year of training causing great and serious inconvenience and waste both of money and time from which the hospital needs protec-

tion. The number of probationers who in the last 7 years completed the
year's training satisfactorily and were transferred to the staff has been 274
out of a total number admitted of 523 thus showing the large number of
249 who for one cause or another relinquished their training.[14]

The high wastage rate is not apparently an inconvenience to the
probationers or to the Fund but to the hospital which relies on their
labour and must be protected. The memorandum goes on to suggest
that a Preliminary Training School on the lines adopted at the London
and Guy's be established at St Thomas's. This document is significant
because the Nightingale Fund report for 1900 stated that

> From the beginning of the School to the end of 1900, 1645 candidates
> have been admitted and 982, after the completion of a year's probation,
> have been placed on the register of Nightingale nurses.[15]

There is no suggestion that the wastage rate had suddenly risen, it
was always round about 40 per cent. The fact seems to be that by the
beginning of the twentieth century the competition for female labour
had intensified, there were other occupations and opportunities for
young women, and nursing was no longer so 'fashionable'. With a
contract to give a three-year service to the hospital the treasurer was
realising that the strength of the main nursing force of the hospital lay
in the retention of the first-year probationers. The hospital was now
calling the tune on nurse training. In 1909 the Fund discussed the
possibility of a Preliminary School. The minutes do not reveal how the
argument went but eventually they agreed with the regulations that
were duly issued in 1910.[16] These stated that the selected candidates
would, before entering the hospital, pass through a six-week course of
instruction, for which a non-returnable fee of five pounds would be
charged. The regulations repeated the undertaking that the successful
candidates would be required to give service to the hospital for four
years after their entry into the Nightingale Home. The salaries showed
little change but the standard of accommodation was improved as the
result of a donation from a governor, and Gaissiot House was opened
in 1906, a further indication of the hospital's interest in the probationers as part of the labour force.

The hospital accepted full financial responsibility for the
Preliminary Training School, which opened in April 1910 under the
supervision of a training sister, and arrangements were made for the
candidates to be examined by Miss Lloyd-Still, a Nightingale nurse, at
that time the matron of the Middlesex Hospital. Before she retired in
1914 Miss Hamilton, the matron of St Thomas's, was able to report
that 'The P.T.S. has been successful in weeding out inefficient and
unpromising pupils and is now beginning to bear fruit with the

numbers discharged steadily decreasing.'[17] The same report stated that 45 certificates had been awarded but it is of interest in showing the changing destination of Nightingale nurses. Sixteen were taken on at St Thomas's and only two went to other hospitals; no less than 27 went into private nursing, an indication that hospitals were training more probationers than they could employ when trained, and the surplus was finding an outlet in the private market.

In 1913 the Court of Governors appointed Miss Lloyd-Still as the matron of St Thomas's. When the Fund Council were told they immediately offered her the post of superintendent of the training school; there is no evidence that the Fund Council was consulted as such but Council members served on the Court of Governors. However, in her absence Miss Lloyd-Still had acquired new ideas about nurse training which she appears to have discussed with the governors before her arrival and these she now proposed to put into action. In March 1914 Miss Lloyd-Still wrote to the Fund Council:

> If you wish to keep educated women for a three year training [sic] it is absolutely necessary that there should be a Sister Tutor separate from the Home Sister (who is now engaged on housekeeping and supervising servants and attending to sick nurses)... [18]

This letter, quoted in the minutes, suggests that the hospital had already agreed to a three-year training and also points to the fact that by now the Home sister was engaged on non-nursing duties and was not fulfilling the function that Miss Nightingale intended. The letter goes on to set out a detailed training programme in which each candidate would do a seven-week course in the Preliminary Training School followed by an examination, after which she would undertake a three-year training during which specific courses of lectures would be given followed by examinations. The other proposed innovation was that gold, silver and bronze medals should be given each year provided that the candidate reached the required aggregate of marks, together with evidence of proficiency. By the time the Fund received these proposals, apparently already in printed form, Henry Bonham Carter was on the point of retiring and his son, Walter, who was to take over the secretaryship, wrote to his father:

> Miss Lloyd-Still's scheme for training and reorganising lectures and appointing a teaching sister has been adopted by the hospital and Miss Lloyd-Still had been authorised to appoint Miss Gullan (now at the Middlesex), and while the hospital hope that the Fund will contribute towards the teaching the hospital would be prepared to find the whole money and Miss Lloyd-Still has been instructed to proceed without waiting for the Fund to come to an agreement.[19]

This letter points up the changed position of the Fund. The hospital realised the value of nurse training, especially if it lasted three years, and they were now prepared, if necessary, to meet all the costs.

Probably most of the Council bowed to the inevitable; however, Henry Bonham Carter did not and said he was sending his criticisms. Unfortunately these are not among his papers, but knowing Miss Nightingale's views on theoretical teaching examinations, a three-year training, badges and medals, they can be guessed. 'Do you not think we are a bit young for the Garter?', she had once quipped to her cousin. However, after 50 years of 'reformed nursing' medicine had changed, as had the health needs of the population, and there was undoubtedly a need for a change in the method of training nurses. Whether a three-year training based on an apprenticeship in an acute general hospital was the best method is a matter for debate.

Whatever their doubts about the new scheme the Fund Council was anxious to retain their controlling interest in the 'probationary year', as the first year was called, and it offered £50 towards Miss Gullan's salary. In the meantime the end of an era had come with the resignation, at the age of 87, of Henry Bonham Carter. In many ways Henry Bonham Carter *was* the Fund and its nineteenth-century history can be traced through the almost daily letters and notes that passed between him and Miss Nightingale, Mrs Wardroper, the Nightingale nurses and the various people with whom the Fund dealt. Although her interest was erratic, while she was alive and active, Miss Nightingale was all powerful in directing the affairs of the Fund, but she soon found her cousin Harry an apt pupil and respected his business acumen. Before long he can be detected taking the initiative. This is apparent in the 'hard bargaining' of 1866, the handling of Mr Whitfield and Miss Barclay, and as early as 1867 he published his own *Suggestions for Improving the Managing of Nursing Departments in Large Hospitals*, which set out the Nightingale system. Soon he was writing authoritatively on nursing matters in medical journals. In 1872 he and four Council members were elected governors of the hospital and Henry became a member of the Grand Council and later an Almoner. He served on many other committees and particularly that cause so near to his heart, the 'National Training for Nurses for the Sick Poor at Home'.

It was not long before Miss Nightingale's letters were peppered with 'Pray advise me' and 'I do not know what to do but to ask you.' Miss Nightingale may have supplied the *bon mot*, but often Henry made the decision. He sorted out the disputes arising from Mrs Wardroper's more arbitrary dismissals, or at least with the probationers who fought back, and one senses that he tried to be scrupulously fair; he poured oil when Miss Nightingale was more than usually censorious, he made arrangements for travel, salaries and postings and personally did much to raise the standard of accommodation that was offered to nurses. Above all, in the troubled days of the 1870s when Miss Nightingale was fearing that 'Mrs Wardroper's mind would turn at any moment', he remained *Ein feste berg*, taking 'the decisions that required calm consideration' without undermining Mrs Wardroper's authority and still retaining her respect. The fact that the Nightingale School survived these storms owes much to his wisdom and his refusal to be panicked into hasty decisions. When asked how he managed to do anything else but serve Miss Nightingale he is reputed to have said, 'When it was getting late I used to say "now I must go home to dinner." '[20]

Before he left Mr Bonham Carter wrote a memorandum on the History of the Nightingale Fund[21] setting out its achievements and laying stress on the variety of its early undertakings, both military and civil, and in particular the Fund's role in laying the foundations of district nursing, an enterprise to which the Fund still made a grant. Now, he pointed out, the Fund had only one liability left and that was to St Thomas's and, since the 'expense for the school was not likely to vary, the Council must now think what to do with their surplus income'. Obviously there was to be no question of giving the whole income to St Thomas's for Mr Bonham Carter went on to stress that:

> Miss Nightingale left no direction to the Council with regard to any new application of surplus income in the objects mentioned by the Trust Deed but it is right that it should be recorded that Miss Nightingale expressed a distinct wish not to be tied to St. Thomas's.[22]

Henry Bonham Carter eventually resigned in April 1914 and at the Council's suggestion his place was taken by his son who was already a member of the Council. Walter was a solicitor with Thorold, Brodie, Bonham Carter and Co. and, having made arrangements with his partners for his salary of £100 as secretary to be paid to the firm to compensate for his loss of time, he accepted, and his place on the Council was taken by his father who remained a member until his death at the age of 94 years in 1921.

At the same time the Council which had shrunk to four was enlarged and further trustees appointed. The policy was, where possible and after permission from the Master of the Rolls, to appoint relatives of the Nightingale family and those closely connected with her original work. The trustees were now the Marquis of Crewe, the son of Lord Houghton, the Earl of Pembroke, the grandson of Sidney Herbert, and Sir Harry Calvert Verney, the grandson of Miss Nightingale's brother-in-law and Viscount Goschen. The Council included, among others, Mr Samuel Shore Nightingale and Mr William Gair Rathbone, the son of William Rathbone.[23]

In 1915 the Fund Council made proposals for a new agreement with St Thomas's Hospital in which they set out the relative financial commitments for the Nightingale School as borne by the Fund and the hospital. The Fund was still paying according to the 1903 agreement which meant that they paid the salary of the Superintendent, the Home sister, the gratuities to teaching sisters, the salaries for 24 first-year probationers and all the lecturing expenses incurred in the first year, all of which came to £930. The hospital was entirely responsible for the Preliminary School, all the training costs for the second- and third-year students, some of the training costs for the first year and all the overhead expenses. The proposal made by the fund was they should pay all the training costs including the Preliminary School while the hospital took over the items that 'were more to the benefit of the hospital such as uniforms and the salaries of the first year probationers'.[24] For some reason those logical proposals were never implemented and there is no evidence as to why not, though a minute many years later suggests that it may have been 'due to wartime circumstances'. This, however, does not account for the fact that no action was taken after the war on what was clearly an anomalous and confusing situation that few people understood.

Before this, early in 1914, the Fund Council set up a sub-committee consisting of Mr Minet, Mr West and Mr Pennard to prepare a scheme, *As to a Postgraduate Course of Instruction for Nurses*.[25] The seven-page report is interesting in the light of the Fund's much later decision to devote its whole income to postgraduate work. The report starts with a brief history of the Fund and the position of nurse training as it was at St Thomas's at that time which suggests that the Council had accepted the three-year training as *de facto* for they write:

> Today a three year training is considered necessary, but in the training given at the St Thomas's School the old plan survives in this way: the training required is three years but the Council only pretends to provide it for the first year during which pupils are called Nightingale Probationers. The two subsequent years' training is undertaken by the Hospital itself.

The report then sets out the conditions for the two classes of candidates and has this interesting note:

> There is no practical difference between the two classes; the reason for the difference is this. The Paying Probationers can obtain a certificate after three years' training, and they are then free to leave, and for many positions it is necessary that they should be able so to leave. The non-

paying Probationers are bound under agreement to serve the Hospital for a fourth year. Their service for this fourth year may thus be considered as a set off against the payment of £30 made by Paying Probationers.

Paying Probationers did not do a 'shorter training' as is sometimes suggested; they were merely let off giving a fourth year of service to the hospital.

The Committee then analysed the expenditure of the Fund and concluded that there would be a surplus income of £550. The questions they had to resolve was how best that money could be spent to further the objectives of the Deed of Trust and would it be desirable to spend more on the Nightingale School itself? In deciding against that course the Committee argued that

> The Nightingale School soon became a model on which other Schools were established... The training of women desirous of becoming nurses is thus amply provided for, nor does the work we do in the Nightingale Home differ today from that being done in other training schools throughout the land.

This being the case the Committee concluded there was no point in spending more money on basic training; the mission in that field was accomplished, instead the Fund should pioneer new fields and that is what Miss Nightingale would have wished. Looking at the new openings for nurses in higher posts the Committee, with great perspicacity, identified the particular shortcomings of the basic training as preparation for higher responsibility. The Committee was in fact echoing Miss Nightingale's complaint, 'We do not train to train'. It was agreed that the best use that could be made of the Fund's money was to fill the gap by providing courses 'dealing with subjects that nurses find painfully lacking'.

In view of the decision taken by the Council in 1974 to spend its whole income on postgraduate training, it is worth quoting the final conclusion of the Committee:

> The condition of the Fund at the present moment would seem to be ideal for an experiment. The existing surplus is sufficient for the purpose and from its success or failure judgement may be reached whether it were wise to enlarge the scheme and to devote to this higher training a larger proportion, *or even the whole income.*

Such a course would involve giving up the present commitment with St Thomas's hospital. Miss Nightingale contemplated this as some day possible, nor is the Fund bound either legally or morally to the hospital. Every hospital has to undertake its own training, and, as things are,

St Thomas's does, as we have seen, undertake the major part of the training of its nurses.

The Committee suggested that as an experiment the surplus income should be used to finance Nightingale nurses in 'courses held at King's College for Women, a branch of the London University that supplies to women higher education in most branches of knowledge'. This then was the position of the Nightingale Fund at the outbreak of the First World War. They were considering opting out of their commitment to the basic training at St Thomas's and spending their income on postgraduate courses for nurses. Counsel's opinion as to the legality of this course was subsequently taken.[26]

How seriously the Council discussed the more radical aspects of the report is not clear, but one thing that militated against the changes was the fact that owing to wartime conditions the courses they contemplated using, which were connected with the University of London, were no longer available and the exigencies of war were such that suitable candidates were not forthcoming. The Fund Council became involved with the Joint War Organisation and this, during the war, absorbed its surplus income.[27] During the war, and after, the association with St Thomas's was strengthened by the appointment of Sir Arthur Stanley, the treasurer to St Thomas's to the Fund Council, and the anomalous joint financial arrangements for first-year nurses persisted until 1937.

However, although the Fund Council remained prestigious its pioneering days were clearly over when Miss Lloyd-Still introduced a three-year training in 1914. Later, when state registration was introduced in 1919 neither the Fund Council nor the hospital authority had complete control of the syllabus or of what were the criteria necessary for a trained nurse.

Today the Fund Council spends its increased income on financing, from any training school, nurses who meet the Council's requirements and who wish to undertake postgraduate work. They are in fact fulfilling the need that Miss Nightingale and Mr Bonham Carter pinpointed a century ago. It remains true that a basic training on the wards of an acute general hospital does not prepare nurses either for supervision of teaching, nor yet for their wider role in meeting the health needs of the population.

Notes

1. Melosh, B., *The Physician's Hand* (Temple University Press, Philadelphia, 1982), p. 32.

2. Abel-Smith, B., *The Hospitals* (Heinemann, London, 1963), p. 148.

3. *Nightingale Fund Council Report*, 1980.

4. H. Bonham Carter to J.G. Wainwright, GLRO, A/NFC/9, 5 September 1891.

5. Ibid., 27 March 1892.

6. Ibid., 17 June 1904.

7. GLRO, A/NFC2/2, 15 May 1902, Minutes.

8. Ibid., 2 March 1903.

9. H. Bonham Carter to J.G. Wainwright, GLRO, A/NFC/9, 24 April 1904.

10. GLRO, HI/ST/NTS/C20.

11. *Memorandum of Instructions by Matron to Ward Sisters on Duties to Probationers*, GLRO, HI/ST/NTS/C17.

12. H. Bonham Carter to H.J. Dudman, GLRO, HI/ST/NC18.31, 19 July 1904.

13. BL, Add Mss 47746, quoted in Clarke-Kenney, A.E., *The London 1840–1940*, vol. 2 (Longmans, Green & Co., London, 1963), p. 123.

14. Memorandum from J.G. Wainwright, GLRO HI/ST/NC18.51 (unnumbered), January 1910.

15. *Nightingale Fund Council Report*, 1900.

16. Regulations for the Preliminary Training School, GLRO, HI/ST/NTS/A2/2, 1910.

17. *Nightingale Fund Council Report*, 1900.

18. A Lloyd-Still to H. Bonham Carter, GLRO, A/NFC/19/1, 26 May 1914.

19. Walter Bonham Carter to H. Bonham Carter, GLRO, A/NFC/9.2, 13 July 1914.

20. Cook, Sir E., *The Life of Florence Nightingale*, vol. 2 (Macmillan, London, 1913), p. 121.

21. GLRO, A/NFC/9, 13 February 1913.

22. Ibid.

23. GLRO, A/NFC/2/2, 9 June 1914.

24. *Proposals for a New Agreement with St Thomas's Hospital*, GLRO, OHI/ST/NTS/AI/6, 3 February 1915.

25. Report of Sub-Committee consisting of Mr. W. Minet, Mr. A.W. West and Mr D.F. Pennant as to Postgraduate Course of Instruction for Nurses (Thorold, Brodie & Co.), GLRO, HI/ST/NTS/A6/1, March 1914.

26. Minutes quoting Counsel's opinion, GLRO, A/NFC2/2, 11 November 1914.

27. GLRO, A/NFC2/2, 19 February 1915.

13. Conclusions

If we examine what the Nightingale School achieved in its first ten years it is in fact very little. A total of 196 names were entered on the register, but these included some who were observers only; of those who signed the contract 64 were dismissed (five for insobriety), while several died either within their training year or in their first post. In the early years, with the exception of Agnes Jones, few made any mark on nursing.

Nevertheless, in spite of this unspectacular beginning, the Fund's experiment was hailed as both revolutionary and successful. Both Miss Nightingale and the Council were indefatigable in their efforts to obtain publicity; they wrote letters to *The Times* and medical journals, Sir Joshua Jebb addressed the Social Science Association, Bonham Carter and Rathbone wrote pamphlets and books and Miss Nightingale herself never missed an opportunity. Agnes Jones's death produced 'Una and the Lion', a straightforward recruiting appeal, and Timothy Daly's death produced *Suggestions on the Subject of Providing Training and Organising Nurses for the Sick Poor in Workhouse Infirmaries*. While Miss Nightingale was writing bitterly to Henry Bonham Carter, 'we have only produced two training sisters' and that Mrs Wardroper was acting like a 'semi insane king', both Mrs Wardroper and the training were being lauded in the press and emulation urged.

Publicity had two effects. First, other hospitals anxious to improve their hygiene, and therefore their nursing, seized on the Nightingale system which they copied whole or in part. The new nurses would improve the cleanliness and hospitals would become safer and more attractive places. Some hospitals overcame the cost by taking a higher proportion of paying probationers who tended to be the better educated, and who, profiting by doctors' lectures, undertook the tasks formerly done by dressers, thus redefining what was the proper task of the nurse. Second, the Nightingale School itself attracted a number of educated and motivated recruits who, paradoxically, sometimes exposed flaws in the training system but who enabled the Fund to start schools elsewhere. Cosseted and coached by Miss Nightingale, backed by the Fund Council and continually advised by Henry Bonham Carter, the group of early 'Specials' started schools in Edinburgh, St Marylebone, Westminster, Birmingham, Wolverhampton and elsewhere. Sometimes the Nightingale influence was short lived and only in Edinburgh did it remain permanently. At St Mary's, Paddington, after the resignation of Rachel Williams, it was left to Miss Medill from the Middlesex to start a training school, and at St Bartholomew's Miss Machin's unhappy tenure was succeeded by Ethel Manson from the London who started a training school in 1877. Curiously, a probationer who *did* make her mark was one whom Miss Nightingale disliked and denigrated, Rachel Strong, who eventually went to Glasgow and started a Preliminary Training School and an improved system of training: Miss Nightingale's confidante at Edinburgh, Frances Spencer, opposed both.

Ironically many of the first favoured few on whom so much advice and exhortation had been lavished married, probably preferring the comfort of a home of their own to the rigours of the Nurses' Home. As widows several started profitable nursing homes, and committed an even greater cardinal sin: they joined the British Nursing Association. The influence of the Nightingale nurses as founders of schools elsewhere is perhaps not so great as the Fund's publicity suggested.[1] There were other runners in the field.

Public recognition enabled the Fund to embark on experiments in other spheres. Perhaps of greatest importance, and least recognised, was the effect of the Fund on Poor Law nursing, first in Highgate, then at St Marylebone, from whence the ripples spread across the pond of Poor Law nursing in general. These experiments did much to ensure that patients in Poor Law infirmaries were eventually nursed by trained nurses. The other field in which the Fund made a great impact was that of trained district nursing. The training programme for the Metropolitan and National Nursing Association was largely planned by Miss Nightingale and Council members and the first district nurses were trained at the Nightingale School, partly at the expense of the Fund. When the Queen Victoria Jubilee Institute for Nurses came into being the Metropolitan and National became the central school for district training, starting a system that continued with comparatively little modification until the National Health Service.

In its official reports the Fund made much of its influence on military nursing.[1] However, in spite of the fact that the Fund trained the early Netley nurses, this area cannot be claimed a success and military nursing pursued its erratic course unheedful of the advice offered by the Fund. Ultimately the main principles were recognised and incorporated into the regulations for the Queen Alexandra Nursing Service, but it is doubtful whether this was directly attributable to Miss Nightingale and the Fund. This has been highlighted by the research of Dr Summers, who points out that at the end of the century doctors were complaining that: 'the whole system of female nursing in the army appears to have been clumsily grafted on to the old system of nursing by orderlies... The graft has never taken root.'[2] Likewise, although reports made much of the effect of the Fund in the Empire, the two main experiments can hardly be counted a success. However, in spite of Miss Osburn's name being deleted by Miss Nightingale, she was probably the main reason for the system being adopted in Australia.

The main contribution of the Fund must be that it brought the concept of secular nurse training into being much earlier than would otherwise have been the case. Sooner or later, scientific medicine and the changed use of the hospital would have brought nursing reform, but the fact that many hospitals resisted the requirements that Henry Bonham Carter thought necessary shows that the idea of training was not universally acceptable in 1860. The publicity of the Fund probably forced the pace of acceptance, and in the end that 'humble experiment' of 1860 became the orthodoxy of 1900.

But is this what Miss Nightingale intended, and was it necessarily beneficial? Was the system set up in 1860 to meet the needs of the sick poor in public hospitals suitable for the changed needs of hospitals in 1900? To what extent had the needs and aspirations of the nursing recruits changed? Miss Nightingale urged 'we must proceed slowly and by experiment' but in the 1890s she had grown old and more reactionary, and with the exception of her interest in public health nursing, she was no longer interested in experiment.

In 1860, when Miss Nightingale aimed her training at those classes in which 'women are habitually employed in earning their living', comparatively few had any formal education. In the ensuing years there had been vast changes; there had been a growth of voluntary schools providing education for women, and in 1870 the Education Act had empowered School Boards to establish schools and to levy a rate to pay for them. By 1865 Cambridge had admitted girls to its local examinations, putting girls, as regards examinations, on equality with the secondary education of boys. The corollary was university education for women. Girton was founded in 1869, then Newnham followed by two colleges at Oxford. The educational background of recruits in 1900 was very different from that of 1860 and their aspirations were different. Learning how 'to pin up checks', wash utensils and obey orders no longer satisfied them, they wanted to know why things were done. As nursing has found since, in order to keep the brighter pupils something more intellectually stimulating was needed.[3] By 1900 the better educated recruits found this stimulus not in developing nursing care but in learning from, and taking over, techniques from the doctors. They became Miss Nightingale's dreaded 'medical women'.

Greater educational opportunities for women, the women's movement and the increase in clerical work created more opportunities for women. By 1901 there were 172,000 women schoolteachers and by 1911 some 51,000 women in the civil service and local government.[4] Although women were still painfully disadvantaged they now had more opportunities, and the more advanced workers in the feminist cause looked with disfavour on nursing because it was women's work dominated by men. Much ink has been spilt on nursing and the women's movement, but strangely enough, with the exception of stalwarts like Mrs Bedford Fenwick and her followers, nurses themselves were little interested in the movement. They had work which most found interesting and which, compared with other women workers, was not as badly rewarded as is sometimes supposed. Comparisons are difficult and there is no doubt that nurses were paid more in kind than in cash. Sometimes the living conditions were good; providing a comfortable Nurses' Home became an important recruitment inducement. Probably compared with an elementary school teacher in the 1870s, who earned £76[5] a year trained nurses were in a better position and, of course, private nursing could be quite lucrative.

However, this was not the main reason why nurses rejected the feminist call to arms. First, most were isolated in a Nurses' Home in what Goffman has called 'the total institution',[6] a place where the social boundaries between private and public life collapsed. Nurses worked, slept, ate, played and prayed together; cut off from friends and families they developed a culture and folklore of their own. Working upwards of a 70-hour week they had little time or energy for anything outside the day-to-day hospital concerns. They did not see themselves as 'dominated by men' but rather by women.

Second, as Dr Summers has shown,[7] nurses had gained status, not only by the improved image of hospital nursing and the Queen's Nurses on the district, but by their participation in the national effort, both in the Empire and in war. During the Boer War and in the frenzied expectancy of war that followed, and the founding of the British Red Cross and the Queen Alexandra Imperial Nursing Service in 1902, nurses had broken into the world of men without trying to displace them. They did not want to be soldiers but they were proud of their military-style uniforms, their badges and their medals. It was a status and prestige that other women workers could not emulate. Florence Nightingale was right when she accused nurses of being conceited. But like her, many thought that they had achieved citizenship without the vote.

Another reason for the lack of interest in suffrage was that many nurses took their cue from the 'ladies' either from within nursing or from those on governing bodies who tended to be wives of establishment figures, to whom 'the women's movement was anathema'.[8] Moreover nurses had it drilled into them that they must be a-political, which generally meant supporting the established order. This was another unfortunate legacy for nursing, though not from Florence Nightingale who was unashamedly radical and would take on half the cabinet to get her way, and who had no qualms about trying to bring the government down. Brian Abel-Smith said that nurses saw 'activism as unprofessional'.[9] He might have added 'unladylike'.

The Nurses' Home with its emphasis on regulations, obedience, Bible classes and chapel twice a day was no longer as appropriate as it had been in 1860. There is no doubt but that some of the high wastage was due to the regulations being out of step with the spirit of the twentieth century.

The second change that would have modified the initial experiment was in medicine itself. The concept of Listerian antisepsis, the validation of the germ theory and the greater use of anaesthesia revolutionised medicine. Once medicine became more scientific nurses needed to understand the reason for the treatment they gave. This need was met by more doctors' lectures, which were often modified lectures for medical students. But probationers were full-time assistant nurses under a contract to do the work of the hospital and theory and practice were not related. Miss Nightingale saw the danger and tried to introduce a 'Mistress of the Probationers' who would teach on the wards, but the idea was resisted by Mrs Wardroper and the hospital authorities. The Nightingale Council was powerless to enforce independent teaching for its probationers.

Since the Nightingale Council agonised over the problems created for nurse training by the contract with St Thomas's the question must be asked whether anything could have been done to change the situation if they had spent capital. Would an independent College of Nursing have been possible? Even if such a scheme had been considered two reasons militated against it. First, there was the lack of trained nurse teachers – there was no 'teacher training College' for would-be tutors. Second, the Council were caught in the web of their own cleverness; they had continually reported the success of the scheme; therefore, why change it? A new scheme would have to be attached in some way to a hospital or hospitals, and there was the question of how much independence the governors would allow. The Fund's probationers were seen by many as a cuckoo in the nest, more independence and a higher academic standard would have been an anathema and seen as a threat to the doctors themselves.

However, the greatest obstacle to change came from the nurses themselves. The Nightingale nurses were reared in an atmosphere of obedience and conformity and the second and third generations clung tenaciously to the principles that had raised them, first to respectability then to admiration. Obedience is inimical to innovation. It is significant that the matrons who came after Mrs Wardroper made no attempt to change the pattern of training; the superintendent of nurse training continued as the matron of the hospital responsible for supplying a nursing service as cheaply as possible. Ironically matrons paid lip-serve to the 'Nightingale system' forgetting that Miss Nightingale had fought, and lost, the battle to give the probationers their own 'Mistress' or Director.

For better or worse the Fund succeeded in carving out an empire for nursing, the matron was supreme in nursing matters and nurses became accountable to nurses. This was not only important managerially, it also gave a career structure, status, and the hope of a reasonable salary within the sphere of women's work. The new nurses were not slow to expand this empire; the way to rise to reward was not through nursing but through layers of superintendence.

The other important legacy of the Nightingale Fund was a system of training based on a working apprenticeship. There is nothing to suggest that in 1860 any other body would have proposed anything different. Paradoxically the system became so popular with hospitals that it remained the orthodoxy for nurse training long after the need for modification had been manifest. Miss Nightingale did not solve the problem and the authorities who took over the responsibility for nurse training did not see the problem and the General Nursing Council, when it came in 1919, fixed the system with legislation.

Contrary to what is supposed Miss Nightingale gave nursing one portal of entry. Her school was open to 'any woman from any class and from any Church', the lady had to be educated with her cook, and she insisted that the training was the same but she wrote 'unquestionably the educated will be more likely to rise to the post of superintendent, but not because they are ladies but because they are *educated*'. This philosophy was acceptable in the class ideology of the 1860s, but the problem arose when society became more egalitarian. Soon the system of Lady Probationers was not one of selecting an élite for matrons' posts but a question of paying money to the hospital to buy a shorter contract.

In the twentieth century, as medicine became more scientific, the question arose as to whether better educated nurses should have a more academic training and education, and, more important, whether that education should be designed to meet the total health needs of the population, not just the sick in the wards of an acute general hospital. For over half a century nursing has agonised over the problem. The enrolled nurse has come and gone, so have at least seven major reports on the education of nurses.[10] The reaction in each case has been much the same; first, it will be too expensive and the service will break down, an argument, if one were needed, of the truth of Florence Nightingale's words that '*our Pros are doing half the hospital's work*'. Second, and sadly, often hostility from those trained in a different system to those entering the profession by another route. Project 2000 students should take heart from the fact that the first Nightingale nurses were resented by the regular nurses at St Thomas's, who often declined to show them anything. The Lady Probationers were resented by the ordinary probationers, because they were supposed to be on a fast track, by virtue of paying. The newly State Registered nurses were often ignored by the unregistered nurses and university graduates from combined trainings were often condemned by doctors and many nurses as being 'unpractical', before they had set a foot in the wards to prove themselves one way or the other. It was ever thus. Historians get a sense of déjà vu.

Medicine has changed and is changing; like Heraclitus's river you cannot step into the same place twice. The large general hospital with its high technology and the rapid turnover in and out of the expensive bed is no place to teach the nursing needs of the whole community. Much of the world of the sick and disabled is elsewhere.

With the coming of antibiotics and the revolutions in surgery nurses lost an empire and had to find a new role. The wheel has come full circle: nurses are now administering and prescribing care, often divorced from the acute hospital, but now this care must be knowledge-based and founded on research. It is a situation that Florence Nightingale would have recognised. She would have welcomed the idea of nurses as independent carers. She, who said 'there is a reason for everything' and complained bitterly about the lack of general knowledge in women, would not, in the light of changed circumstances, have been shocked at the idea of university trained nurses. She, after all, instituted a training for health visitors in technical colleges a hundred years ago. She also wrote: 'I look to the abolition of all hospitals and workhouse infirmaries. But no use to talk about the year 2,000.'[11]

Within the terms of its reference, the Nightingale Fund Council met as best it could, the nursing needs of the 1860s. For 40 years or so it managed to achieve a great deal in various spheres and because of its publicity and prestige, its influence was probably out of proportion to its achievements. The Council was not able to adapt nurse training to the changed needs of the twentieth century, although it is significant that it eventually proposed spending its money on postgraduate education because its income was not enough to pay for the numerous probationers now required to do the work of St Thomas's. Paradoxically the very popularity of the system in economic terms for hospitals was the death knell to its influence. For the next 80 years or so many hospitals were able to staff their wards mainly with students, with wastage at the rate of 30 per cent a year. This is not what Florence Nightingale intended.

Notes

1. *Nightingale Fund Council Annual Report*, 1910 and *Special Report*, 1886.
2. Summers, A., *Angels & Citizens* (Routledge & Kegan Paul, London, 1988), p. 97.
3. *The Lancet Commission on Nursing* 1932, *The Interdepartmental Committee on Nursing Service*, 1937 *The Nursing Reconstruction Committee*, 1942–9 and *The Working Party on the Recruitment and Training of Nurses*, 1947.
4. *Report of the Census of England and Wales* (HMSO, London, 1911).
5. Maggs, C.M., *Origins of General Nursing* (Croom Helm, London, 1983), p. 55.
6. Goffman, E., *Essays in the Social Situation of Mental Patients and other Inmates* (Double Anchor, New York, 1961); see also Melosh, B., *The Physician's Hand* (University Press, Philadelphia).
7. Summers, ibid., p. 7ff.
8. Ibid, p. 27f.
9. Abel-Smith, B., *A History of the Nursing Profession* (Heinemann, London, 1960).
10. Baly, M.E., *Nursing and Social Change*, 3rd edn. (Routledge, London, 1991).
11. FN to H. Bonham Carter, BL, Add Mss 47714, 4 June 1867, f. 203.

Select Bibliography

Primary Sources

Held at the Greater London Record Office (GLRO): *The Nightingale Collection* (the Nightingale Training School), HI/ST/NTS, and *The Nightingale Collection*, HI/ST/NC; *The Nightingale Fund Council Records* (GLRO), A/NFC; *St Thomas's Hospital Records*, HI/ST

Held at the British Library Department of Manuscripts: *The Nightingale Collection*, Additional Manuscripts 43394, 45750–45754, 45774, 45784–45788, 45792–45796, 45800, 47714–47723, 47726, 47738, 47739, 47759.

Held at Wilton House: the *Herbert Papers*, vols. 1855–61.

Held at the Wellcome Institute for the History of Medicine: Selected extracts of the Nightingale letters on microfiche including selections from the *Claydon House Papers*

The Middlesex Hospital Archives: the *Nursing Records*, vols. 1855–70; *Committee Reports*, 1860–70

Secondary Sources

Reports and Government Publications: *The Third Report of the Select Committee on the Metropolitan Hospitals* (HMSO, London, 1892); *The Select Committee on Registration of Nurses* (HMSO, London, 1904); *Census of Population 1871, 1901; The Inter-departmental Committee on Nursing Services* (Athlone), Interim Report (HMSO, London, 1939); *The Nursing Reconstruction Committee* (Horder) Four Reports; *The Royal College of Nursing 1942–9; The Committee of Nursing* (Briggs) (HMSO, London, 1972)

Journals

The Nursing Record, 1889-92; *The Lancet* 1866–8, 1888–9; *The Nursing Mirror*, 1897—1910; *The Nursing Times*, 1908–10

Pamphlets and Articles

Bonham Carter, H. (1867) *Suggestions for Improving the Management of the Nursing Department in Large Hospitals* (Blades & Blades, London)
— (1888) *Is a General Register for Nurses Desirable?* (Blades & Blades, London)
Hall, Mrs Carter S. (1861) 'Something of What Florence Nightingale Has Done and Is Doing', *St. James's Magazine* vol. 1. (April) pp. 29–40
Lückes, Eva, C.E. (1889) *What will Trained Nurses Gain By Joining the British Nurses' Association?* (London), pamphlet

Writings by Miss Nightingale

Letters Written by Florence Nightingale in Rome in the Winter of 1847-1848) (ed. Keele, M.) (American Philosophical Society, Pennsylvania, 1981)
Female Nurses in Military Hospitals (Panmure Papers, 1857) (Hodder & Stoughton, London, 1908)
Subsidiary Notes as to the Introduction of Female Nursing in Military Hospitals in War and Peace (Harrison & Sons, London, 1858) presented by request to the Secretary of State for War
Notes on Nursing: What it is and What it is Not, 2nd edn (Harrison and Sons, London, 1860)
Suggestions for Thought to the Searchers after Truth among the Artizans of England, 3 vols. (Eyre and Spottiswoode, London, 1860), privately printed
Notes on Hospitals, 3rd end (almost completely rewritten in 1863) (Longmans, Green and Co., London, 1863)
'Suggestions on the Subject of Providing Training and Organising Nurses for the Sick Poor in Workhouse Infirmaries' in *Report of the Committee on Cubic Space of Metropolitan Workhouses*, 19 January 1867, pp. 64–9
'Una and the Lion', *Good Words*, June 1868
Introductory Notes on Lying-in Hospitals, together with a Proposal for Organising an Institution for the Training of Midwives and Midwifery Nurses (Longmans, Green & Co., London, 1871)
Addresses to the Probationer Nurses in the Nightingale Fund School at St Thomas's Hospital, 1872-1900. Printed for private circulation
Letter to the Nurses of the Edinburgh Royal Infirmary, 1878. Printed for private circulation
On Trained Nursing for the Sick Poor (Spottiswoode & Co., London, 1881), pamphlet
History of District Nursing, 'A History of Nursing in the Homes of the Poor' Introduction by F. Nightingale in a book by William Rathbone dedicated to Her Majesty on the foundation of the Queen Victoria Jubilee Institute (Macmillan, London, 1890)
In a *Dictionary of Medicine*, R. Quain (ed.), 'Nurses, training of', and 'Nursing the Sick' (Longmans, Green & Co., London, 1882), reissued 1910, pp. 1038–43; 1043–9

An invaluable guide to Miss Nightingale's writings is *A Bio-Bibliography of Florence Nightingale*, compiled by W.J. Bishop and completed by S. Goldie (Dawsons, London, 1962)

Books

Abel-Smith, B. (1960) *A History of the Nursing Profession*, London: Wm. Heinemann

— (1964) *The Hospitals: 1800-1948*, London: Wm. Heinemann

Ayers, G.M. (1971) *England's First State Hospitals, 1867–1930*, London: Wellcome Institute for the History of Medicine

Baly, M.E. (1997) *A History of the Queen's Nursing Institute*, London: Croom Helm.

— (1995) *Nursing and Social Change, 3rd edn*, London: Routledge.

— (1987) *'As Miss Nightingale Said...* , 2nd edn. London: Baillière Tindall

Battiscombe, G. (1974) *Shaftesbury – Biography of the 7th Earl*, London: Constable

Boyd, N. (1982) *The Victorian Women Who Changed Their World*, London: Macmillan

Branca, P. (1975) *The Silent Sisterhood*, London: Croom Helm

Briggs, A. (1954) *Victorian People*, London: Pelican

Cadbury, M.C. (193) *The Story of a Nightingale Nurse*, London: Hedley Bros.

Calabria, D., Macrae, J. (1994) *Suggestions for Thought – Selections and Comments*, Philadelphia PA: University of Pensylvania Press.

Cameron, H.C. (1954) *Mr Guy's Hospital*, London: Longmans, Green & Co.

Chadwick, O. (1970) *The Victorian Church, Part 1 & 2*, 2nd edn., London: Adam & Charles Black

Clarke-Kennedy, A.E. (1963) *The London 1840–1940*, London: Longmans, Green & Co

Collins, S. (1995) *A Brief History of the Royal London Hospital*, Royal London Hospital Archives & Museum.

Cook, Sir E. (1913) *The Life of Florence Nightingale*, 2 vols., London: Macmillan

Cope, Z. (1955) *A Hundred Years of Nursing at St. Mary's Hospital, Paddington*, London: Wm. Heinemann

— (1958), *Florence Nightingale and the Doctors*, London: Museum

Crow, D. (1971) *Victorian Women*, London: Allen and Unwin

Dacre Craven, F. (1889) *A Guide to District Nursing*, London: Macmillan

Davies, C. (ed.) (1980) *Rewriting Nursing History*, London: Croom Helm

Donnison, J. (1977) *Midwives and Medical Men*, London: Wm. Heinemann

Fischer, R.B. (1977) *Joseph Lister 1827-1912*, London: MacDonald & Janes

Garmarnikov, E. (1978) 'The Sexual Division of Labour: The Case of Nursing' in A. Kuhn & A.M. Wolfe (eds), *Feminism and Materialism: Women and Modes of Production*, London: Routledge & Kegan Paul

Goldsmith, M.L. (1937) *The Woman and the Legend*, London: Hodder and

Stoughton

Goodman, M. (1862) *The Experiences of an English Sister of Mercy*, London: Smith, Elder & Co.,

Hálevy, E. (1932) *The History of the English People*, vols. IV and VI. *The Victorian Years and the Rule of Democracy*, London: Earnest Benn

Hector, W. (1973) *Mrs Bedford Fenwick*, London: Royal College of Nursing

Herbert, R.G. (n.d.) *Florence Nightingale – Saint, Reformer or Rebel*, New York: Robert R. Kreiger Publishing Co.

Hodgkinson, R.S. (1967) *The Origins of the National Health Service, the Medical Services of the New Poor Law 1834–1871*, London: Wellcome Historical Medical Press

Humble, J.C. and Hansell, P. (1974) *The Westminster 1716–1974*, London: Pitman Medical Press

Huxley, E. (1975) *Florence Nightingale*, London: Weidenfeld & Nicholson

Iremonger, L. (1958) *Lord Aberdeen (Prime Minister 1852–55)*, London: Collins.

Jones, A.E. (1872) *A Memorial to Agnes Jones by her Sister*, London, Strahan & Co.

Jowett, B. (1987) *'Dear Miss Nightingale' A selection of letters Benjamin Howett to Florence Nightingale 1860-1893* Ed Vincent, Q. & Prest, J. Oxford: Oxford University Press

Kamm, J. (1965) *Hope Deferred: Girls' Education in English History*, London: Allen & Unwin

— (1966) *Rapiers and Battleaxes – The Women's Movement and Its Aftermath*, London: Allen & Unwin

Lambert, R. (1963) *Sir John Simon 1816–1904*, London: MacGibbon & Kee

Laslett, P. (1965) *The World We Have Lost*, New York: Methuen

Longford, E. (1964) *Victoria, R.I.*, London: Pan

— (1981) *Eminent Victorian Women*, London: Weidenfeld & Nicholson

Lückes, E. (1886) *Hospital Sisters and Their Duties*, London: Churchill

Maggs, C. (1983) *The Origins of General Nursing*, London: Croom Helm

Maggs. C.M. (Ed.) (1987), *Nursing History The State of the Art*, London: Croom Helm.

Mayhew, P. (1987) *The Birth & Growth of a Community*, Oxford: Parchment.

Medvei and Thornton (eds) (1974) *The Royal Hospital of St Bartholomew's 1123–1953*, Ipswich: W.S. Cowell

Melosh, B. (1982) *The Physician's Hand*, Philadelphia: Temple University Press

Moore, J. (1988) *A Zeal for Responsibility: the Struggle for Professional Nursing in England*, University of Georgia.

Myers, P. (1996) *Building for the Future – A Nursing History from 1896–1996 to commemorate the centenary of St Mary's Convent, Chiswick*, Chiswick: St Mary's.

Nutting, M.A. and Dock, L.L. (1907) *A History of Nursing. The Evolution of Nursing Systems from the Earliest Times to the Foundation of the First*

English and American Training Schools for Nurses, New York: G.P. Putnam's Sons

Oliver, B. (1966) *British Red Cross in Action,* London: Faber.

O'Malley, I.B. (1931) *Florence Nightingale 1820-1856),* London: Thornton Butterworth

Osborne, H. and Godolphin, S. (1855) *Scutari and Its Hospitals,* London: Dickinson & Brothers

Parsons, F.G. (1936) *The History of St Thomas's Hospital,* 3 vols., London: Methuen

Peet Van, R. (1995) *The Nightingale Model of Nursing,* Edinburgh: Campion Press.

Piggot J. (1975) *Queen Alexandra Army Nursing Corps,* London: Leo Cooper

Pope-Henessy, J. (1949–52) *Monckton Milnes – The Years of Promise 1809–1850.* The Flight of Youth 1851–1855. London: Constable

Rathbone, E. (1890) *William Rathbone: A Memoir,* London: Macmillan & Co.

Rathbone, W. (1890) *Sketch of the History and Progress of District Nursing,* London; Macmillan & Co.

Ridley, J. (1970) *Lord Palmerston,* London: Constable

Saunders, H. St G. (1949) *The Middlesex Hospital 1745–1948,* London: Max Parish

Seymer, L.R. (1960) *Florence Nightingale's Nurses 1860–1960,* London: Pitman Medical Pess

Smith, F.B. (1982) *Florence Nightingale – Reputation and Power,* London: Croom Helm

Stanmore (Lord Gordon, A.H.) (1906) *Sidney Herbert: A Memoir,* 2 vols., London: John Murray

Stratchey, L. (1948) *Eminent Victorians,* London: Penguin (Chatto & Windus edn: 1918)

Strocks, N. (1960) *A Hundred Years of District Nursing,* London: Allen & Unwin

Summers, A. (1988) *Angels and Citizens British Women as Military Nurses 1854–1914* London: Routledge & Kegan Paul.

Tooley, S. (1910) *The Life of Florence Nightingale,* London: Cassell & Co.

Verney, H. (ed.) (1970) *Florence Nightingale of Harley Street,* London: Dent (1968) *The Verneys of Claydon,* London: Robert Maxwell

Vicinus, M., Negaard, B. (1989) *'Ever Yours Florence Nightingale',* London: Virago Press.

Watson, F. (1911) *The History of the Sydney Hospital 1811–1911,* Sydney: Gullick

Wheatley, V. (1957) *The Life and Work of Harriet Matineau,* London: Secker and Warburg

Willis, I.C. (1931) *Florence Nightingale,* London: Allen & Unwin

Woodham-Smith, C. (1960) *Florence Nightingale,* London: Constable

Webb, R.K. (1969) *Modern England,* London: Allen & Unwin

Yeo, G. (1995) *Nursing at Barts.* Stroud, Glos: Alan Sutton Publishing Ltd.

Youngerston, A.J. (1979) The Scientific Revolution of Victorian Medicine, London: Croom Helm

Unpublished Theses

Felgate, R.V.R. (1977) 'The Emergence of Militancy in the Nursing
    Profession', PhD thesis, University of Surrey
Granshaw, L.P. (1981) 'History of St Thomas's Hospital, London
    1850–1900'; 'Noble and Womenly Work', from PhD thesis, London
    University
Prince, J.E. (1982) 'Florence Nightingale's Reforms of Nursing 1860–1877',
    PhD thesis, University of London

APPENDIX I – Example of a Nurse's Personal Record Sheet

Layout of the Red Register to be filled in by Miss Wardroper and counter signed by the Resident Medical Officer

| Name of Probationer | By whom recommended | Nature of duty during the year $\Big\}$ | No. of days | Time off duty from illness during year $\Big\}$ | Days |
| | | | No. of nights | | Hours |

| Age at last birthday preceding her appointment $\Big\}$ | Names of Sisters under whom she has served $\Big\}$ | | | Nature of such illness* $\Big\}$ | |

Single or married, or widow   Religion

Date of appointment

MONTHLY STATE OF PERSONAL CHARACTER AND

Underneath the following Five Heads, state the Amount of Excellence or Deficiency, under the Three Degrees, "Excellent," "Moderate," "O".

	1. PUNCTUALITY. Especially as to administration of food, wine and medicine	2. QUIETNESS.	3. TRUST- WORTHINESS.	4. PERSONAL NEATNESS AND CLEANLINESS.	5. WARD MANAGEMENT (or Order.)
January					
February					
March					
April					
May					
June					
July					
August					
September					
October					
November					
December					

*

continued.

	6. HELPLESS PATIENTS. Moving. Changing. Personal cleanliness of. Feeding. Keeping warm or cool. Preventing and dressing bed sores. Managing position of.	7. BANDAGING. Making bandages. Making rollers. Lining of splints, &c.	8. MAKING BEDS. Removal of sheets.	9. WAITING ON OPERATIONS.	10. SICK COOKING. Gruel. Arrowroot. Egg flip. Puddings. Drinks.
January					
February					
March					
April					
May					
June					
July					

APPENDIX I – Example of a Nurse's Personal Record Sheet (cont.)

August
September
October
November
December

+

*If defective, state nature of defect in this line.

MORAL CHARACTER DURING PROBATION

SOBRIETY*   HONESTY   TRUTHFULNESS
                          (Especially as to taking petty
                          bribes* from patients)

*In each of these Columns state the Nurse's character (from the experience of
the year or of any shorter period, if dismissed: positively; no degree admissible;
the first dereliction ensures her dismissal.

ACQUIREMENTS OF NURSE DURING HER PERIOD OF SERVICE.

The Following Degrees are to be used in each Monthly Entry:– "Excellent" – "Good" –
"Moderate" – "Imperfect" – "O'."

1. DRESSING. Blisters. Burns. Sores. Wounds. Fomentations. Poultices. Minor dressings.	2. APPLYING LEECHES. Externally. Internally.	3. ENEMAS. For men. For women.	4. MANAGEMENT OF TRUSSES, AND UTERINE APPLIANCES.	5. RUBBING. Body. Extremities.

+

11. KEEPING WARD FRESH. By night. " day.	12. CLEANLINESS OF UTENSILS. For cooking. " secretions	13. MANAGEMENT OF CONVALESCENTS.	14. OBSERVATION OF THE SICK. Secretions. Expectoration. Pulse. Skin. Appetite. Intelligence as delirium, stupor. Breathing. Sleep. State of wounds.	GENERAL REMARKS. Eruptions. Formation of matter. Effect of diet, stimulants, medicines, Signs of approaching death.

+ State in this line any duty in the columns in which the Nurse is prominently excellent (E.)
or imperfect (I.)

APPENDIX II

The Diary of a Special Probationer in 1890

7.00 a.m. Went on duty. Helped the night nurses' side; washed two patients

7.30 Helped on the day nurses' side; washed a convalescent patient

8.00 Went to prayers

8.15 Washed a typhoid patient

8.30 Washed the urine bottles and the locker tops with chlorinated soda

8.45 Washed and dusted Sister's table and the window ledges. Cleaned and trimmed the lamps. Washed the urine and medicine glasses and small jugs …

9.15 Prepared the lunch – bread and milk, served it round

9.45 Went into the bathroom: washed out bath, basins and traps. Put fresh cloths on the ice bowls, folded and put away the clean mattress. Tidied the pillow basket

10.15 Went off duty

11.00 Went to Sister's class

12.45 p.m. Went to dinner

1.30 Came on duty. Made beds with Nurse Chaplin. Washed the wine glasses, dusted and tidied the centre of the ward.
Put ready the dressing gowns for the doctor

1.50 p.m. Cut up 7lbs of beef for beef tea – made beef tea

2.20 Attended Dr Ord's round and waited on Sister

3.15 Went to Steward's office with a telegraphic message

3.30 Helped Sister to wash an unconscious patient

4.00 Filled three steam kettles

4.20 Cut thin bread and butter for fever patients, prepared tea, served tea round, fed a patient

5.50 Came off duty (tea, 25 minutes)

6.15 Went on duty. Washed specimen glasses, washed feeders, washed gas globes, gave patients their supper

7.15 Made the beds with Nurse Moon

7.45 Tidied the Centre. Arranged and lighted the lamps. Arranged the ink stands. Took out the flower pots. Turned down the gas

8.00 Carried round the wines and brandies

8.15 Collected the wine glasses

8.30 Came off duty

8.45 Went to prayers

9.00 Had supper

9.20 Went to bed

APPENDIX III Nightingale Nurses – 1860–1868
An Analysis of what Happened to the First Nightingale Nurses, data copied from the Register 1860–1868

ENTERED TRAINING: JULY 1860 – JULY 1861

Reg. No.	Name	Age	Status	Health in Training	Training Report	Appointments (Contract) 1861–62	1862–63	1863–64	Subsequent Career
1.	Mary Barker	32	S	Sore throat	Good	S.T.H. trans Netley. Liverpool Work Ho. Inf.			1867 Sister Sydney Hosp. NSW; ret. Edinburgh in 1876
2.	Jane Couchman	30	S	Sore throat	Good	S.T.H. (nurse) Liverpool Inf.		No further mention ? disappeared (no gratuity)	
3.	Annie Lees	33	S	Sore throats	Good		S.T.H. trans Liverpool Work Ho. Inf. (left ill-health)	Rugby School (left ill-health)	
4.	Emily Medhurst	25	S	Septic finger	Deficient in nicety	Bath (left – 'no-one knows where')			
5.	Marie Mullion	24	S	–	DISMISSED – DISOBEDIENCE				
6.	Martha Murdoch	31	S	Pulmonary Infection	DISMISSED – ILL HEALTH (?TB)				
7.	Susan Newman	29	S	–	DISMISSED – INSOBRIETY				
8.	Charlotte Nixon	31	S	–	Good – exceedingly good in all duties	Liverpool – DIED – TYPHUS (soon after arrival)			

No.	Name	Age	S/W	Illness	Conduct	Service / Appointments	Notes
9.	Harriet Parker	25	S	Typhoid & scarlet fever	Generally good	Sick S.T.H. – left the Service	
10.	Mary Phillips	29	S	Jaundice bronchitis	Good	Warrington Work Ho. Inf. – ? (no further info.)	
11.	Georgina Pike	29	S	Hysteria, sore throat	V. good – reported lectures well	S.T.H. S.T.H. S.T.H.	?Left the service
12.	Elizabeth Stephens	29	S	RESIGNED			
13.	Caroline Stone	22	S	Scalds, sore throats	V. good	Bath Bath (Matron) Bath (Matron)	Matron R.U.H. Bath
14.	A.M. Tennant	40	W		DISMISSED – DISOBEDIENCE		
15.	Emma Whitlock	34	S	Scarlet fever	Not strong enough, not educated	S.T.H. S.T.H. – LEFT – ILL-HEALTH	

ENTERED TRAINING: JULY 1861 – JANUARY 1862 (thereafter Register January to January)   Appointments (Contract) 1862-63   1863-64   1864-65

No.	Name	Age	S/W	Illness	Conduct	Service / Appointments	Notes
16.	Fanny Wilde	30	S	Sore throat	Good	S.T.H. – MARRIED	
17.	Sarah Terrot	32	S	Sore throat, diarrhoea	Good	RESIGNED	
18.	Elizabeth Perrottie	30	S	Sore throat, fever	Somewhat opinionated	S.T.H. Leicester Infirmary (Head Nurse) Devonport Hospital	
19.	Ann Reilly	29	W		DISMISSED – INSOBRIETY		
20.	Elizabeth Bane	40	W		DISMISSED – INCOMPETENT		

Reg. No.	Name	Age	Status	Health in Training	Training Report	Appointments (Contract) 1862-63	1863-64	1864-65	Subsequent Career
21.	Mary Hind	34	W	Hepatitis, scarlet fever	Fairly good	Edinburgh Royal Infirmary	DISMISSED – FORGETFUL		
22.	Helen Terrot	31	S	Returned to St John's House (special arrangement) to help with teaching spelling and reading (Came to St. Thomas's)					
23.	Rebecca Riggott	32	S	Typhus, sore throat	Good	S.T.H./Nottingham/Woolwich Mil. Hosp.		Norwich Gen. Hosp.	
24.	Margaret Garson	29	S	Typhus	Good	Liverpool W.H. Inf.	Devonport	?	
25.	Elizabeth Cox	35	S	Bronchitis	Excellent		S.T.H.	Addenbrookes (Sister)	
26.	Deborah Burgess	34	S	Inflammation	Good leg and foot	S.T.H.	MARRIED		
27	Harriet Shooter	34	S		DISMISSED – INEFFICIENT				
28.	Fanny Huston	35	S	Debility	Not strong enough	DIED – TYPHUS			
29.	Jane Squires	37	S		Good	S.T.H. Dorset Country	MARRIED		
30	Annette Martin	29	S		Excellent	S.T.H.	S.T.H.	S.T.H.	Becomes Sister 'Extra'. Subject of FN's bitter attacks Left 1872

No.	Name	Age	S/W	Illness	Assessment	1863	1864	1865
31.	Anabelle Hickman				DISMISSED – UNSUITABLE			
32.	Susan Hickman	31	S		DISMISSED – UNSUITABLE			
33.	Ellen Powell	30	S	Typhus	Good plain nurse	Liverpool Inf.	Liverpool	RESIGNED
34.	Elizabeth Wotton	26	S	Typhus	Good plain nurse	S.T.H.	S.T.H.	Addenbrookes (Sister)
35.	Elizabeth Kilovert	34	S		DISMISSED			

ENTERED TRAINING: JANUARY 1862–1863

No.	Name	Age	S/W	Illness	Assessment	Appointments 1863	1864	1865
36.	Henrietta Walker	34	S	Neuralgia, influenza	Good	Kings College	Liverpool Inf. (Nurse)	DIED 1921
37.	Mary Merryweather	41	S	Only 2 months as a 'pupil' (sent by Mr Rathbone)		Lady Supt. Royal Inf. Liverpool		
38.	Eliz. Merryweather	37	S	Only 2 months		Ass/Lady Supt. Royal Inf. Liverpool		
39.	Emily Markham	23	S	Sore throat	Good, well informed	Cardiff Infirmary (Matron)		
40.	Fanny Lovesay	33	W	Hepatitis debility	Good, superior education	Guys	Gen. Hospital, Salford (Matron)	
41.	Mary Piety	33	S	Sore throat	F./good	DISMISSED – INDISCRETION OF CONDUCT TOWARDS STUDENTS		
42.	Agnes Jones	29	S	Deafness, debility	Excellent	Supt, Northern Hospital Work Ho. Inf.	Lady Supt Liverpool DIED TYPHUS 1868	

Reg. No.	Name	Age	Status	Health in Training	Training Report	Appointments (Contract) 1863	1864	1865	Subsequent Career
43.	Betty Lillycrapp	33	S	Sore throat	Good	S.T.H.		Northampton Gen. MARRIED	
44.	Helen Oliver	35	S		DISMISSED – IMPROPRIETY		?ALCOHOLISM, DRUG ADDICT		
45.	Harriet Turner	23	S		DIED OF SCARLET FEVER – BURIED AT NORWOOD AT THE EXPENSE OF THE N.F.C.				
46.	Ann Batchford	31	S	Debility Chest infec.	DISMISSED – POOR HEALTH				
47.	Caroline Blowman	24	S	?Phthisis	DISMISSED – POOR HEALTH				
48.	Margaret Wilkes	29	W	Debility	DISMISSED – POOR HEALTH				

ENTERED TRAINING: JANUARY 1863–1864

Reg. No.	Name	Age	Status	Health in Training	Training Report	Appointments 1864	1865	1866	Subsequent Career
49.	Anna Hearne	27	S	Billious	Satis. Poss. of making a good nurse	S.T.H./Liverpool	Liverpool Work Ho.	County Hosp. Dorchester (Head Nurse)	
50.	Fanny Beardmore	31	S		Good	S.T.H.	Liverpool Work Ho. Inf. (Head Nurse)	Liverpool	Not listed again
51.					MISSING				
52.	Nora Kennedy	27	S		DISMISSED – MORAL CHARACTER DEFECTIVE				
53.	Mary Sales	37	S		DISMISSED – INSOBRIETY				
54.	Hannah Frenfield	27	S		Very good	S.T.H.	Liverpool Work Ho. Inf. (Head Nurse)		

No.	Name	Age	S/W	Complaint	Character	Appointments			
						1864	1865	1866	
55.	Mary Chalcroft	25	S	Colds	Satisfactory	S.T.H. MARRIED			
56.	Mary Chapman	27	S	Inflammation of the legs	Satisfactory	S.T.H. MARRIED			
57.	Mary Trueman	26	S	Headache	Satisfactory industrious	S.T.H.	Liverpool Work Ho. Inf	Liverpool	Middlesex Hospital DISMISSED, UNFIT FOR SISTER'S POST
58.	Mary Snow	30	S		DIED OF TYPHOID				
59.	Emma Flood	35	W	Colds	Good	S.T.H.	Liverpool Work Ho. Inf	Liverpool	
60.	Elizabeth Trueman	29	S		Good	S.T.H.	Liverpool Work Ho. Inf	Liverpool	Middlesex Barts (Sister) DIED 1920
61.	Elizabeth Harvey	27	S	Hysteria Haemorrhagia	Fair/good	Sick	S.T.H./ Liverpool Work Ho. Inf.	Liverpool	Middlesex Hosp. DISMISSED UNSUITABLE
62.	Ann Tissington	24	S	Phthisis	DISMISSED – POOR HEALTH				
63.	Maria Inwood	35	W	Typhus	Good	S.T.H.		Liverpool	DISMISSED

ENTERED TRAINING: JANUARY 1864–1865

#	Name	Age		Illness	Rating	Appointments 1865	1866	1867
64.	Susan Jeans	24	S	Rheumatism Chest condition	Excellent	Liverpool Work Ho. Inf.		
65.	Ann Burgess	32	W	Erysipelas and fever	Good	Liverpool Work Ho. Inf.	DISMISSED	
66.	Ann Duffey	28	W	Colic	Good	S.T.H.	S.T.H.	S.T.H. MARRIED
67.	Emily Bull	29	S	Poisoned finger, fever	Good	Liverpool Work Ho. Inf	Liverpool	S.T.H. (Sister)
68.	Emma Wilkington	41	Sep		DISMISSED AFTER A MONTH			
69.	Angela Burcheur	36	Sep		DISMISSED			
70.	Leonara Biscoe	39	S	Cold	Good	Addenbrookes	DISMISSED	
71.	Mary Silver	30	S	Sore throat Poisoned finger	Good	Stafford Inf.	Dorset County	Liverpool Hosp. Inf. Diseases (Matron)
72	Lucy Emm	32	S	Cold Sore throat	Good	Liverpool Work Ho. Inf.	Liverpool Work Ho. Inf.	Netley (Head Nurse) — Left Netley 1876 – DISMISSED
73.	Marion Bradbury	24	S		A fair nurse	S.T.H.	Cardiff Inf.	DIED
74.	Ann Blundell	27	W	Neuralgia	Moderate abilities	S.T.H.	Winchester	S.T.H. (Sister Adelaid)
75.	Louisa Francis	31	W	Billious	RESIGNED			

No.	Name	Age		Illness	Temperament	Appointments		
						1866	1867	1868
76.	Sarah Dexter	29	S			Bradford (Matron)	RESIGNED – ILL HEALTH	
77.	Elizabeth Foster	23	S	Sore throat	Moderate	S.T.H. (Nurse)	Manchester N. Assoc.	
78.	Matilda West	27	S		A fair nurse	S.T.H.	Derby Inf. MARRIED	

ENTERED TRAINING: JANUARY 1865–1866

No.	Name	Age		Illness	Temperament	1866	1867	1868
79.	Anna Henna	32	S	Fever Sore throat	Good nurse	S.T.H.	Lincoln County	DISMISSED
80.	S. Coulthord	29	S	Colic	Moderate	Manchester N. Assoc.		
81.	Mary Wayte	30	S	Good	MARRIED			
82.	Elizabeth Walton	30	S	Rheumatic fever	Good	Manchester N. Assoc. for Hospital Workers	Manchester	
83.	Sarah Henderson	33	S	Sore throat		Manchester N. Assoc.		
84.	Mary Brieley	37	S	Erysipelas	Good	Manchester N. Assoc.		
85.	Ellen Cullen	27	W	Colds/cough	Good	S.T.H. (nurse)	MARRIED	
86.	Agnes Lindsey	29	S	Accident Chest Inf.	F. good	S.T.H.	Margate Inf.	Invalided
87.	Mary Rehnolds	24	S	Fever Sore throat	Moderate	S.T.H.	Winchester Inf.	MARRIED
88.	Emma Clark	24	S	Fever	Good plain nurse	S.T.H.	Derbyshire County Hosp.	MARRIED

Reg. No.	Name	Age	Status	Health in Training	Training Report	Appointments (Contract) 1866	1867	1868	Subsequent Career
89.	Mary Mackie	33	S		Excited, nervous	Manchester N. Assoc.			
90.	Ellen Rigley	34	S	Colds Billious	Good	S.T.H.	S.T.H./Swansea		
91.	Alice Hubble	31	S		A plain nurse No particular ability	S.T.H.	Swansea (Head Nurse)		
92.	Jane Bishop	21	S			S.T.H.	Winchester Inf.	DISMISSED	
93.	Elizabeth Blundell	26	W	Neuralgia	Plain nurse Good	S.T.H.	S.T.H.	Sydney Hosp New South Wales	DISMISSED
94.	Mary Farrell	20	S	Rheumatism	Moderate ability	S.T.H.	S.T.H./B.R.		
95	Ellen Dawtrey	33	W		Good	Margate Inf.	MARRIED		
96.	Betty Chaunt	28	W	Sore throat	Very good	S.T.H.	Derbyshire County	Sydney Hosp. New South Wales	DISMISSED
97.	Charlotte Wood	39	S	(Only 5 mths training)	Well educated Conscientious	Hampstead Union Superintendent	RESIGNED		
98.	Elizabeth Goddard	33	W	Fever/cold	Ordinary capacity	S.T.H.			
99.	Mary Ward	33	S	Hepatitis	Intelligent Good nurse	S.T.H. (Sister)	DISMISSED FOR INSUBORDINATION, SOBRIETY DOUBTED		

						Appointments		
	ENTERED TRAINING: JANUARY 1866–1867					1867	1868	1869
100.	Jane Markham	26	S	Neuralgia	Intelligent (Only 8 mths)	Swansea (Matron)		
101.	Mary Gregory	26	W	Cold	Good plain nurse	S.T.H./ Derbyshire County Inf.	RESIGNED	
102.	Mary Barber	30	W	Colds	Good plain nurse	Lincoln County Inf.	RESIGNED	
103.	Annie Miller	32	S	Colds Sore throat	V. industrious Excellent surgical nurse	Derbyshire /Sydney Hospital County Inf. / New South Wales		DISMISSED
104.	Annie Baster	34	S		Fair nurse	S.T.H. (Sister)	S.T.H.	
105.	Florence Lees	25	S		Well educated Fair surgical nurse	(Did very little training; did not comply with regulations)		1874 Super/ Met. Nursing Assoc. Later – Mrs Dacre Craven
106.	Elizabeth Young	31	W	Colds	Useful Intelligent	Netley/S.T.H. (Did part of training at Netley)	Devonport	
107.	Mary Bratstone	44	W		Good – part at Netley	Union Hampstead	Hampstead	
108.	Mary Whitton	39	S	Operation for tumour	A person of mod. capacity	Lincoln/S.T.H.	Blackburn (Matron)	
109.	Emma Rappe	31	S		Well educated lady (8 mths only)	Returned to Sweden – Matron in Uppsala		

Reg. No.	Name	Age	Status	Health in Training	Training Report	Appointments (Contract) 1867	1868	1869	Subsequent Career
110.	Elizabeth Kilvert	38	S	Cold/cough	5 mths training only	Derbyshire County (Lady Superintendent)			
111.	Helen Turriff	32	S	Cold	Good, intelligent	Sydney Hospital New South Wales (Sister)		DISMISSED	
112.	Mary Clark	35	S	Sore throat	Very good	S.T.H.	S.T.H.	Netley	
113.	Mary Hart	34	S	Cold Sore throat	Plain nurse	S.T.H.	S.T.H.	S.T.H.	
114.	Mary Butler	25	S	?Glandular fever/Irites	An intelligent nurse/good ability	S.T.H.	S.T.H.	S.T.H.	FN calls her 'an evil influence'
115.	Lucy Osburn	29	S	Intermittent fever	Lady of superior birth Mistress of several languages	Sydney Hospital, New South Wales (Lady Superintendent)			Stayed in NSW
116.	Frances Smith	26	S		LEFT AFTER 4 MONTHS				
117.	Clara Cullen	26	S	Sore throat	RESIGNED				
118.	Isabella Trydell	22	S	Cold	DISMISSED ON DISCLOSING SHE HAD ENGAGEMENT WITH ONE OF THE PORTERS				
119.	Mary Reeves	25	S	Scarlet fever	Good	S.T.H.	Winchester Country Hosp.		
120.	Elizabeth Chung	25	S	Febricula	?	S.T.H.	Winchester County Hosp.	MARRIED	

No.	Name	Age	Season	Illness	Assessment	Outcome / Appointments
121.	Jane Williams	30	S			DISMISSED – UNSUITABLE
122.	Sarah Townsend	22	S	Scarlet fever		DISMISSED – NOT STRONG ENOUGH FOR THE WORK
123.	Charlotte Money	31	S	Infection of foot		DISMISSED – NOT STRONG ENOUGH FOR THE WORK
124.	Anna Reeves	33	W	Cold Sore throat	Plain nurse Moderate	Derby County
125.	C. Mottram	38	Sep		Incompetent	DISMISSED
126.	Ann Sullivan	38	W	Gastric derangement	Truthfulness doubtful	Blackburn (Head Nurse)
127.	Ann Nash	29	S	Cold	Moderate nurse	S.T.H.
128.	A.R. Jones	31	S	Debility	Good	?

ENTERED TRAINING: JANUARY 1867–1868

No.	Name	Age	Season	Illness	Assessment	Appointments		
						1868	1869	1870
129.	Lucy Kidd	31	S	Tonsillitis	Very good, exemplary character	Liverpool (Lady Superintendent)	DISMISSED – MISCONDUCT	
130.	Lucy Stabler	30	W		Fairly good	S.T.H.	S.T.H.	S.T.H.
131.	Sarah Nash	32	S		DISMISSED – REFUSED TO SIGN AGREEMENT			
132.	Mary Thomas	32	S	Sore throat	Fair ability Industrious	Gloucester Inf. (Superintendent)		
133.	Harriet Elleman	41	S	Cold	RESIGNED – NOT STRONG ENOUGH			

Reg. No.	Name	Age	Status	Health in Training	Training Report	Appointments (Contract) 1868	1869	1870	Subsequent Career
134.	Catherine Collins	29	W	Sore throat	Moderate abilities (mainly 'goods')	Derbyshire Inf. (Head Nurse)	DISMISSED – DISOBEDIENCE		
135.	Rebecca Strong	23	M	Cold	Good practical nurse	Winchester	Netley	Netley	Matron, Glasgow Started 1st PTS 1880
136.	Martha John	20	W	Febricula	?	S.T.H.	MARRIED		
137.	Julie Abbot	26	S		DIED OF TYPHOID				
138.	Emma Berry	32	S	Cold	Fair nurse	S.T.H.	S.T.H.	Netley	Head Nurse Edinburgh 1876
139.	Harriet Saunders	26	W		DISMISSED				
140.	Jane Duke	37	S	Sore throat	Superior person	S.T.H. (Sister)	S.T.H.	MARRIED	FN called her a bad influence
141.	Margaret Westle	32	S	Cold	Good	S.T.H.	S.T.H.	Edinburgh	
142.	Amelia Harris	42	S	Rheumatism	Plain nurse	S.T.H.	RESIGNED		
143.	Sarah Trueman	44	S	Fever	6 mth training	Matron at Winchester – special arrangement			
144.	Mary Winsall	35	S	Cold Sore throat	Fairly good	S.T.H.		Netley	

				RESIGNED – NOT STRONG ENOUGH FOR THE WORK
145.	Sarah Litchfield	26	S	Febricula	
146.	Henrietta Somerville	38	S		A lady of good ability	RESIGNED – NOT WILLING TO CONFORM WITH REGULATIONS
147.	Catherine Tyrell	35	S	Colds	No comment	S.T.H. ADMITTED AS A PATIENT TO BETHLEHEM ASYLUM
148.	Elizabeth Montforte	23	S	Colds	A woman of moderate ability	MARRIED

Index

247